LIVE
BEFORE
YOU
DIE

FRANS HUMAN

ISBN: 1461169747
ISBN-13: 9781461169741

You might ask: "Why this title? Of course I shall live before or until I die." However, the real question to ask yourself is: "Am I really living, or do I merely exist?"

None other than Helen Keller said: "Life is either a daring adventure or nothing."

The purpose of this book is to show older people that life can still be a daring adventure regardless of your age.

Indeed, (old) age is no excuse not to live life to its fullest.

That is what this book is all about. You'll find many practical guidelines and invaluable advice in this book. You only have one life on this earth and for all the older people, time is quickly running out. The good news is that you can do something about still living a quality life. The bad news is only you can make it happen.

I hope I meet you between the pages of this little book. It is a little book with big rewards.

This book is dedicated to my wife Gerda who is assisting me to practice what I preach, and to Frans, Jan-Louis, Narina, Henk, Tanya, and die vier karnallies Chanè, Luan, Luca, and Maya.

It is also dedicated to older people who refuse to use age as an excuse not to live life to its fullest.

Mynderd Vosloo illustrated this book. Thank you, Mynderd, for doing a sterling job. The illustrations are great!

INDEX

CHAPTER 1

LIVE BEFORE YOU DIE

This book is written with the older people in mind. Please note that I am referring to "older" people and not the "elderly." I honestly do not know for which age group this book is intended. There is no law or rule book that states at what age a person is to be regarded as old or elderly. Even our nation's constitution, which is quite an extensive document, says nothing about when a person is to be regarded as old. One gets a young fifty-year-old and an old fifty-year-old. You'll find an old eighty-year-old and a young eighty-year-old. What then, if we are not talking about a specific age group, are we talking about?

We are talking about older people. More specifically it is about older people who think they are too old to live life to its fullest. For all of you older people who do not live life to its fullest, this is your wakeup call!

A wise man once said, "God, you have lots of time—I don't. Help me to live before I die." This piece of wisdom, which should be everyone's prayer, was shared with the world in a poem by Father Frans Claerhout.

1

Claerhout was also a very famous and prolific painter and his paintings have been exhibited across North America, Belgium, Canada,Germany and, of course, South Africa.

Let us repeat Father Claerhout's piece of wisdom: "God, you have lots of time—I don't. Help me to live before I die." This book is all about the idea that we shall live before and until we die. That may sound very obvious to you. Surely we shall all live until we die. However, the question is do we really live until we die, or are we merely existing—going on day after day without a purpose in life. The excuse we frequently use is that we are too old to do exciting things. We are too old to live a meaningful life.

What utter nonsense!

None other than Helen Keller said, "Life is either a daring adventure or nothing". The purpose of this book is to show elderly people that life can still be a daring adventure regardless of your age.

I know too many people who are thinking and acting like elderly people while they still could enjoy a higher quality life. I know too many people who allow society to consider them old because they have reached a certain age. May I repeat, there is no rule to determine when you are old. In fact, old age has no age limit!

I also have the impression that too many of my fellow senior citizens are merely sitting in the sitting room or in front of the television set just waiting for death to come.

This reminds me of the story about four friends in a retirement village who regularly played a hand of bridge. The person who always organized the card game was William. Two members of the foursome were John and Gareth. John and

Gareth were next-door neighbors and would always arrive together. One day John arrived without Gareth. "Where is Gareth," William asked. "Is he ill?" John replied, "No. Gareth says he's too old to play bridge, and he is just sitting in front of the television set." William asked, "But why is he just sitting in front of the television set?" John answered, "I don't know. I think he is waiting for death to come." So William said, "Go tell Gareth to get off his butt and run until death catches up with him. And he better do it immediately because I want to deal the cards."

We have a choice and we can decide whether we shall still enjoy a quality lifestyle. We can either sit and wait for death to come, or we can get off our butts and go for it. Granted, it depends a lot on our health and whether our minds are still functioning properly. I appreciate that your health and mind could become a challenge. But for the rest of us, get off your butts and go for it.

One thing is true: age should be no hindrance to leading a meaningful life. There is nothing in the rule book that says that age could keep you from living life to the fullest. Age should not be an excuse to stop living fully before we die.

What is a quality life for one person is not necessarily a quality life for another. Whatever your definition of a quality life is, that is what you should pursue. Make the mind shift right now and simply make the decision to live until you die. The idea is that within the limits of the health of body and mind, we shall live a meaningful life regardless of our age. Age is a number. It is a measure of how many years have passed since birth. Not much more than that. Age is also relative. Victor Hugo said, "Forty is the old age of youth. Fifty is the youth of old age."

Mark Twain said, "Age is an issue of mind over matter. If you don't mind, it does not matter."

When my grandfather was fifty-five years old, he stopped farming actively, and sat on the verandah drinking lots and lots of coffee. The community of that time regarded a man of fifty-five to be an old man. The community had literally made my grandfather an old man. Even worse, my grandfather also believed this and agreed with the community. The result was an old man at the age of fifty-five. What a waste!

Yes, I know I cannot hit the golf ball as far as I used to, but I can still actively participate in golf games and competitions, and enjoy it. I hit the golf ball a shorter distance but more accurately and in that way still maintain an acceptable golf handicap.

Psychologically it is true that once you decide you are too old for an activity, lo and behold, you *are* too old for that activity. Do not fall into this trap, and more importantly, do not allow anyone else to make that decision for you.

I am not naive and I know that there will come a day when physically you won't be able to manage, but until that day, go for it.

With the increased and effective health care that is available these days, people are unquestionably living longer than before. If these extended years are also coupled with good health, the quality of life is so much better. Good mental health care is as important as good health care for the body.

The combination of good bodily and mental health care would surely influence your lust for life and your perception of old age. In the context of the message of this book, your perception of old age is vitally important and has an enormous effect on your lifestyle.

The tendency to lower the retirement age all the time is really a crime against older people. Originally the retirement age was sixty-five, then it was lowered to sixty, and then even to fifty-five years. What is even more disturbing is that this is happening in a so-called developing country where there is an acute shortage of skills and where competent human resources are a luxury. How organizations can argue that people of fifty-five and over cannot still make valuable contributions is simply unthinkable. It is indeed in those years that you still can be very productive at the work place and apply the valuable experience you have gained over many years.

In the United States this ridiculous practice is not followed, and you find people in key positions who are much older than people in senior positions in South Africa. While the expertise of older people overseas is effectively applied, a developing country like South Africa does the opposite and then complains about the lack of sufficient expertise and qualified people! The solution to the problem is obvious.

There are many examples of people who are already far beyond the "normal" retirement age and can still make a great contribution. A good example in this respect is Alan Greenspan, the chairman of the Federal Reserve of the most powerful country in the world. Various presidents of the United States, including Ronald Reagan, George H.W. Bush, and Bill Clinton, appointed Dr. Greenspan. George W. Bush also appointed Greenspan as chairman of the Federal Reserve. At that point, Alan Greenspan was already seventy-eight years old! It was not about whether Dr Greenspan was past "normal" retirement age. It was about Greenspan's proven expertise and competency in his field. This should be the only criterion.

In the next chapter we shall meet a few (there are many more) older people who did not use old age as an excuse not to excel in their field of expertise. What springs to mind is "God, you have lots of time—I don't. Help me to live before I die." This is exactly what these people did, and what you and I should do.

After meeting with these great people, we shall also look at some very practical issues that can assist us in leading a quality life. If we still have a meaningful purpose in life, it can be the reason why we would want to get up in the morning with great expectancy of what is lying ahead.

Other important matters we will address are:

- You can do something about your weakening/ deteriorating memory;
- Exercise that brain;
- Taking those pills;
- Money matters;
- Your last will;
- Driving your car;
- Contracts and agreements;
- Exercise and social life;
- You must (still) have a purpose in life;
- Personal hygiene.

On the last pages of this book there will also be a summary of the essence of each chapter. Use these as a checklist to ensure you are on track to live until you die.

While living until you die, it is important not to lose your sense of humor. Your memory could fail you at times, and you will get into awkward situations that are sometimes also hilariously funny. Also see the funny part of it. Even enjoy what seem to be smaller embarrassments. As Oscar Wilde puts it: "Life is too important to be taken seriously."Life is too serious to be (only) serious about life. Older people might not have lots of time to live life to the fullest. Don't miss out on this opportunity!

CHAPTER 2

AGE IS NO EXCUSE

When one looks at the achievements of older people all over the world, one thing is very clear: You are never too old to do what you really want to do. You are never too old to pursue your realistic dream!

These people truly lived and will live before they die. They do not sit waiting for death to come. They did not and are not using their (old) age as an excuse not to follow their dream. They live life as an exciting adventure.

There was a man of ninety years who married a woman of thirty. She went to the doctor whilst her husband stayed at home. Very excited she phoned her husband. When he answered the phone she said, "Guess what, I am pregnant with your child!" To which her ninety-year-old husband responded, "Pregnant? Who is speaking?"

These people who are really living until they die, don't they also have aches and pains when they get up in the morning? I would not know as these people would normally not concentrate on their aches and pains. I suppose they also have mornings when it is more difficult to get out of bed than other mornings. The issue is not whether they had aches and pains.

The important issue really is that these people have a reason to get out of bed. They want to get out of bed to pursue their dreams!

We have a friend, Bessie Viljoen, who was eighty years old when she published her first storybook for little children. She also did the illustrations herself. Another friend was seventy-two years old when she got her bachelor's degree from a well-known university. She was an ordinary housewife living on a farm in the Karoo in South Africa and had this dream. She simply followed her dream and attained this degree.

Wally Hayward was one of South Africa's top athletes. You can read much more on the enigmatic Wally Hayward on www.wally.org.za. He represented South Africa at the Commonwealth and Olympic Games and held various world records for long-distance running. Wally would later become even more famous for his participation in the Comrades Marathon that annually takes place in South Africa. For me, his most amazing achievement was completing this tough ultramarathon in nine hours and forty-four minutes when he was seventy-nine. And just to show it was not just a fluke, Wally did it again the next year! Wally won the Comrades Marathon for the first time when he was twenty-one years old. This means that he completed the marathon fifty-nine years later! What an achievement and an inspiration for older people!

Let us put this incredible achievement in perspective. The Comrades Marathon is considered one of the most difficult and toughest ultramarathons in the world. This marathon is run over a distance of ninety kilometers (or sixty miles) over a hilly terrain between Pietermaritzburg (inland) and Durban (on the coast) in South Africa. One year the athletes would run down from Pietermaritzburg and the next year the athletes would run up from Durban.

An amazing woman is Dr Bettie Cilliers-Barnard described as the doyenne of South African artists and has become a legend in her time. Bettie Cilliers-Barnard was born on 18 November 1914 in South Africa; at age ninety-five she was still a prolific painter. Dr Cilliers-Barnard has an impressively long list of awards from local and foreign organizations. Amongst these are awards from the International Biographical Center of Cambridge in the United Kingdom and a World Decoration for Excellence by the American Institute (Biographical). She also received three honorary doctorate degrees including one from the University of Pretoria at the age of eighty-eight! In the same year she received another of the many awards she received during her lifetime. This time it was the Prestige Award for Painting from the Thswane University of Technology.

Equally amazing was Anna Mary Robertson who was born in Greenwich, New York, on 7 September 1860. She would later marry farm worker Thomas S. Moses. Little did anybody know that she would become the famous Grandma Moses. She lived on the farm and embroidered pictures in yarn. At the age of seventy-six, because of arthritis, she was forced to give up embroidery. She could, however, hold a brush in her hand, so Grandma Moses started painting. Four years later she held her first solo exhibition in New York City in 1940. This means she was then eighty years old! Clearly this woman was not going to use her age as an excuse not to follow her dream. Two years later Grandma Moses held her second solo exhibition in New York, and as the saying goes the rest is history. She became world famous and would be described as the most famous American folk artists of the twentieth century.

When he died in 1996, the actor George Burns was 100 years old. If one looks at the life of Burns, also described as the legendary American vaudeville comedian, it is clear that

George Burns truly lived until he died. George (his real name was Nathan Birnbaum) lost his wife when he was regarded an elderly person. After his wife's death, he had this running joke of being a sexy senior citizen as he was often seen in the company of beautiful young women. He said he would love to go out with women his age, but there is no woman his age.

George Burns appeared in many movies, in radio and on early television. It is an impressive list of shows and films. What is even more impressive is what happened when he returned to films after an absence of almost forty years. He co-starred with Walther Matthau in Neil Simon's hit *The Sunshine Boys* at the age of seventy-nine and won an Oscar for the best supporting actor! When George Burns won the Oscar, he commented, "It could not have happened to an older guy." When George was eighty-three years old he played a role of an elderly person in *Going in Style*. About his role in this film, George said that he had to learn how to act old. Although this was meant as a joke, I also believe that he was serious about this—such was his attitude toward old age. George never lost his sense of humor. On death he commented, "I can't afford to die. I'd lose too much money."

George Burns' words "It could not have happened to an older guy" were not entirely true as it happened to an older woman. Jessica Tandy received an Academy Award for best actress for her performance in *Driving Miss Daisy* in 1989, when she was eighty years old! When one reads the biography of this talented British-born American actress, one gets the impression that Jessica lived her life to the fullest. When she was eighty-one years old, Jessica was chosen by the readers of *People* magazine "as one of the fifty most beautiful women in the world in 1990."

There is so much to be said about this famous woman. Tandy had an acting career spanning some sixty-five years. About

Jessica it is said that Jessica found latter-day movie stardom in major-studio releases and intimate dramas alike." *Camilla* (1994) was to be her last performance, and it was bold in one way that she, at the age of about eighty-five, had a brief nude scene.

The last thing I would like to advocate is nudity (especially at that age), but what I would like to accentuate is that Jessica Tandy did not use old age as an excuse not to follow her dream.

George Burns and Jessica Tandy are, as far as I know, the oldest people to win Academy Awards.

Another person that we should really take note of is Hans-Georg Gadamer. He was born in Marburg, Germany, on February 11, 1900 and died when he was 102 years old. Gadamer was the author of a large number of books. Most probably the best-known book written by this philosopher was his monumental work *Wahrheit und Methode*, which was published in 1960.(Wahrheit und Methode: Grundzuge einer philosophischen Hermeneutik, Tubingen, Mohr 1960). In this great work, Gadamer gave us an insight on how to interpret art and philosophies based on centuries-old facts. In this book he also explains the (now famous) conflict between truth ("Wahrheit") and methods ("Methode"). Gadamer's approach gave us also new insight in the way we would interpret fine arts and theology. Gademer's goal was to uncover the nature of human understanding.

Apart from his many works on hermeneutics, Gademer is also known for a long list of publications on Greek philosophy and his work on Plato. His last publication that I am aware of was published at the age of ninety-six! (*Der Anfang der Philosophie, Stuttgart, Philipp Reclam*, 1996.) What an incredible philosopher. At the age of ninety-six he could still make a meaningful contribution to mankind. Again we find a man who did not use age as an excuse not to live life to its fullest.

In the autumn edition of *Holidays* of the RCI group Africa there appeared a thought-provoking article titled "Gallivanting Granny" by senior citizen Doris Drummer. Doris decided to join the SKI (Spend the Kids' Inheritance) Club and requested her local travel agent to make reservations for her for an extraordinary trip. She did not tell anybody what she was planning to do. I suppose that was to avoid her children and friends telling her she was too old for such an adventure. Doris' first stop was the Parthenon in Greece, then to Croatia (as she knew nothing about their history), and then she was off to Dubai, the shopping capital of the world. Next she traveled to Australia and the Great Barrier Reef. She took a resort course on scuba diving and went scuba diving on the great reef! Still she was not ready to return home and flew to Brazil and went to the Amazon what Doris described as a another jaw-dropping experience. Her last bit of insanity was a visit to the Grand Canyon, where she took a helicopter trip into the canyon. If that was not enough, Doris figured she got so far why not go north east to Colorado and do some snowboarding—and that was exactly what she did.

I could not find out Doris's real age, but Doris Drummer concluded her story with these words "Age is an attitude, and I'm glad I decided to change mine. Shouldn't you?"[1]

There is a saying "act your age". If Doris had told her children and friends about her plans, they would most probably have advised her to act her age. If there is one saying we older people should erase from everyone's vocabulary, then it must be

---

1 Doris Drummer, Holidays RCI Group, *Autumn* (2010): 33

this one. Act your age? Who decide how one acts at what age? Where is the rule book? Who makes these rules? There are no laws or regulations that prescribe what you should do at what age. Simply ignore this nonsense. You determine the rules for this. You will decide what it really means to act your age.

You always wanted to write that book, you always wanted to do that painting, or you always wanted to publish those poems. If you are ninety-six years of age or younger, you can still do it. Gademer did it and left an important legacy.

"Write, paint, sculpt, learn the piano, or take up dancing. Whether it's the tango or line dancing, start a college course, fall in love all over again—the possibilities are limitless for you to achieve your private ambitions." Joan Collins, actress and writer. [2]

Referring back to the trips of Doris Drummer, I am not advocating that you spend all your money on around-the-world trips. That might not make sense. It is for this reason that I have also included a talk about money matters in this book.

What I am advocating is that you can still follow your dream regardless of your age. It does not matter what your dream is. Again there are no rules or lists of requirements. All that matters is that you must have a dream! It is because we are older that we have to follow our dream—now. Time is running out on us. I really think it is very appropriate to ask the Almighty to help us to live until we die.

To repeat Doris Drummer's words: "Age is an attitude, and I'm glad I decided to change mine. Shouldn't you?"

---

2 Shelly Klein, *The Little Book of Senior Moments* (London: Michael O'Hara Books, 2008),70.

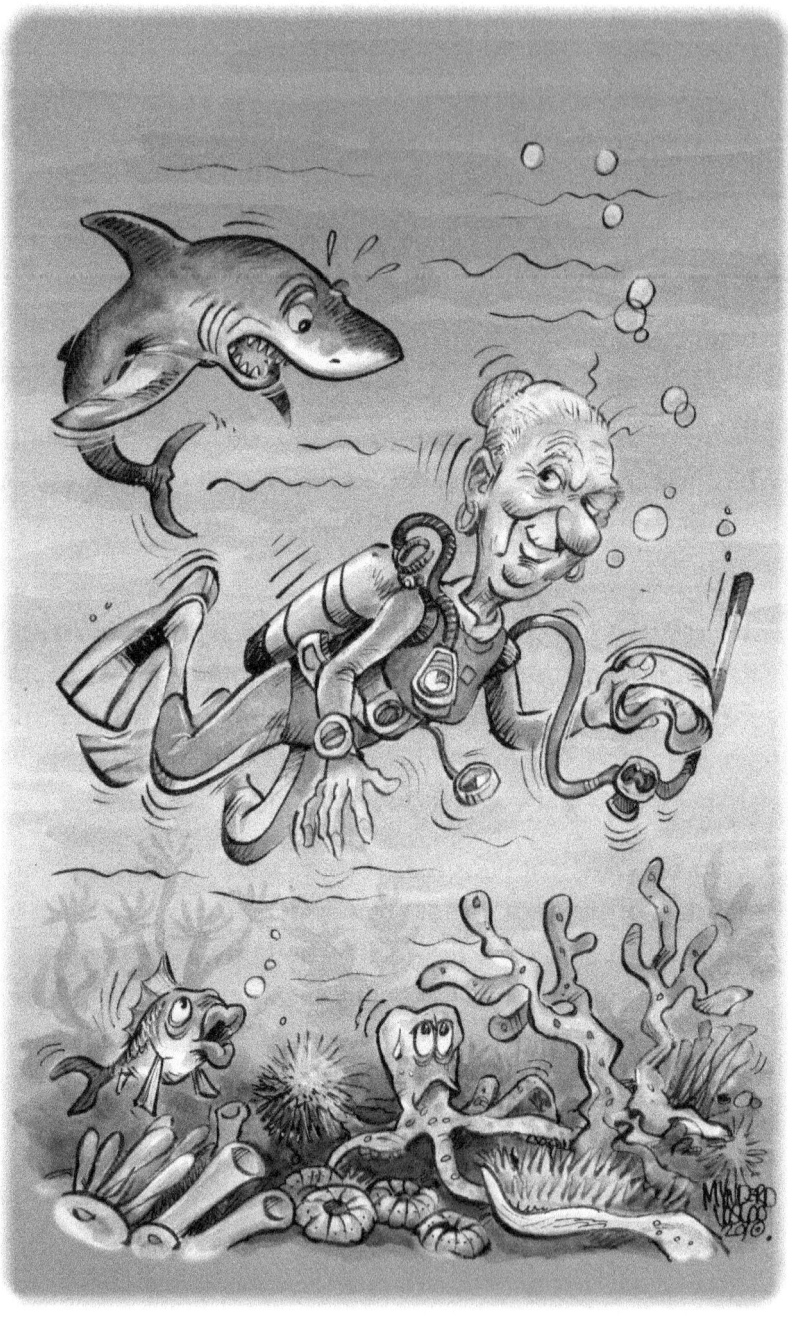

CHAPTER 3

YOU CAN DO SOMETHING ABOUT YOUR MEMORY

Many senior citizens are complaining that their memory is no longer as good as it used to be. Not only that, but their memory seems to get worse as the years march on. (I think some of them forgot that their memory was not so good when they were younger.)

Be it as it may, you can definitely do something about your memory! You can do a number of practical things that will definitely help you in this situation. Yes, you can do something about your memory if you are really serious and want to do something about it. There are many good reasons why you really should make the effort to improve your memory.

A friend tells the following story as to why he does everything in his power to improve his memory. (I heard a similar story on the golf course). He said one day he found an old man sitting on a bench in a park crying bitterly. My friend walked up to this old man and asked, "Why are you crying? Can I help you?" The old man did not respond. "Is it your wife that made you cry?" my friend asked. The old man replied, "No not at all. I am married to a young woman, and she is the best there can be. She cooks me the nicest meals. When I get home she would bring me my slippers and take off my shoes. She gives me all the tender loving care anybody can ask for." My friend asked, "Then why are you crying?" The old man answered, "I forgot where I live."

We might not forget where we live, but we tend to forget many other ordinary things that are really annoying. You know the feeling: You walk to a cupboard to fetch something, but when you get to the cupboard, you do not know why you are there in the first place. You walk upstairs to get something, only to get upstairs and not remember why you went up the stairs. You had a pen in your hand a moment ago when you made a note, but now you do not know where you put the pen. The pen is simply gone. Where on earth are my car keys? I had it in my hand a while ago. Now they're gone. Even worse: I have parked my car in a multistory parking garage. I was pretty sure that I would be able to find my car quite easily that is why I did not make a note of the number of the parking space. Now my mind seems to be a blank, and I can just simply not remember where I parked my car.

I really cannot remember whether I took my medicine or not. For safety's sake I'll take the medicine again. After a while, I am not even sure whether I took all the medicine the second time round. You have hidden your jewelry in a safe place because you are afraid someone might steal it. Congratulations, you've done well. Your jewelry is so well hidden that even you cannot find it.

You did not want to make a note when you lent one of your favorite books to a friend, as you were sure you would not forget who borrowed this book. And you did remember for the first week or two. However, as time went by, it became more difficult to remember until eventually you had no idea who borrowed your book. What is worse, nobody returns the book. There is also the other side of the same coin. There is an older person who borrowed this fantastic book from somebody. It was a great book, and now this person wants to return the book to its rightful owner. The only problem is that this person cannot remember from whom he got this book. Your name and phone number is not written in the book. The result is that you have lost one of your favorite books and somebody is sitting with a book that person would like to return to its owner.

So we can carry on and on.

It is said that a postgraduate student did research on how senior citizens spend their time in an old age home. The results were surprising or perhaps not that surprising. Almost all of the respondents came up with the same answer: We spend most of the day looking for lost stuff. This means that older people are looking for their stuff instead of doing things they really like or care for. What a waste of time and what a waste of life! The worst is still to come. It turned out that after (and if) they found their stuff they put it in a place where they are absolutely sure they won't have to look for it again. But what happens after a week or two? They start looking for the same stuff again. It is like a vicious circle and they cannot get out of it.

In this chapter we would like to look at practical ways in which to dramatically reduce the time you are looking for your stuff. Hopefully you will then have more quality time to live life to its fullest. It is not necessary to waste many hours searching for your stuff. There are simple and practical solutions to improve your memory.

When I did a search on the Internet on how to improve your memory I got around 124 million answers! No, this is not a printing error. There were more than 124 million responses. The responses were varied and very interesting.

Some of the responses:

- "Improve memory with scientifically designed games"
- "Healthy nutrition and supplements that improve memory"
- "Memory with mind tools"
- "Proven system to dramatically improve memory"
- "Memory techniques"
- "Improve memory now".

There were thousands more. If you have some time on hand it can be really interesting to search the Web on this subject.

It is clear that there are thousands of ways and many thousands of experts who are of the opinion that you can improve your memory. I agree wholeheartedly with these people that we can improve our memory. We need not take expensive courses to achieve this.

Years ago I saw an advertisement in our local newspaper on how you can develop a mega memory in a very short period of time. It was offered at a very low price and as I was curious to see what methods they use, I bought the package. When the course material came, I opened it and had a look at the principles they used. I never really had the intention to do the course.

About a year later I had a call from a lady from this "memory company." She asked me whether I bought the memory course a year ago and whether I would be willing to answer some questions. I said I would, and she warned me we were on a speakerphone and that other people in the room would be able to hear our conversation. I had no problem with that and asked her who the other people in the room were. To which she replied they were invited quests. I immediately knew that this was a sales pitch, and I decided to have some fun.

She asked me whether there was an improvement in my memory after I have worked through the memory course. To this I said, "I don't know. I can't remember." There were a few moments of silence before she said, "We have so many positive responses and amazing results of people who took this course." To this I responded, "What course?" Now there was a deafening silence and then, before I could stop her, she quietly put down the phone.

Of course there is nothing wrong with taking a course to improve your memory. Anything goes to help us to improve our memory.

Fortunately there are also other ways to improve your memory and you can even have fun with it. Let's look at very simple techniques to improve your memory. You will be amazed by the results!

Here are some of the basic techniques:

- Keys (when you are at home): The following apply to all keys, car keys, keys to all the doors in your home, the outbuildings, tool boxes, and whatever keys you have. This also applies to remote controls. Always hang or keep your keys in the same place without exception. Always in the same place. The test is this: if there is a power failure in the middle of the night, would you be able to get out of bed and walk straight to where you keep your keys and be able to find any specific key you are looking for? If you cannot do this, your system is not working and has to be looked at again.

  Always wear your keys on your person. This should preferably be in the same place or in a specific section of your handbag or in the same pocket of your trousers. Never put your keys on the counter of the shop or on the table at the restaurant or on the table in a waiting room. Always keep your keys on your person, and you will save hours looking for your keys.

- Glasses (spectacles): Especially when you retire at night, always put your glasses in the same place. Again there should be no exception to this rule. If you think it is difficult to find something that is lost with your glasses, it is nigh impossible to find something without your glasses.

- Cell phone (mobile phone): How many times did you not know where you put it? If at all possible, carry it on your person, especially if you move around. This should preferably be in the same place or in a specific section of your handbag or in the same pocket of your trousers. Have you ever experienced the situation when a cell phone rings, and the lady with the big bag starts unzipping and looking through section after section in her bag? Of course, as soon as she finds the cell phone, it stops ringing. Never put your cell phone on the counter of the shop or on the table at the restaurant or on the table in a waiting room. Always carry the phone on your person. (There are people who think this could be a health hazard, but that is a discussion for another time.) The cell phone charger can also get lost very easily. Always store it in the same place with the power plug you would normally use.

- Backup of the data on your cell phone: If you have any data on your cell phone it is important to backup the data on a regular basis. All the equipment and programs you need to do this normally come with the cell phone and the handbook is normally very clear on how to do it. Do not shy away from this; do the back up, it is fun and a nice accomplishment it if you are generally scared of computers. If you are still reluctant to do this, ask your four-year-old grandchild. They seem to know how to do this type of thing from birth.

- Medication: Medication may only be stored in a safe place and out of reach of children. There cannot be any excuse for not doing this. Make it a habit to put your medication back in the safe place after you have used it. Remember to get your chronic medication before the present batch is finished. There is a whole chapter on medication. It is important that you read it.

- Cameras, binoculars, and similar equipment: Again the golden rule is to store it at a specific location. I also try and keep the battery chargers, computer, and video connections, data cables, memory sticks, and tapes of each camera together. I store them together, so that the specific camera with all its peripherals are easy to get to. You might also want to keep the manuals and handbooks at the same place. If everything is stored together, it makes it easier and more fun to use.

- Sport equipment: Sport equipment should also be stored at a specific location. I like to keep all the stuff I need for that specific sport together. With my fly-fishing equipment, I also keep my rods, extra line, flies, and even the priest together. If you would invite me for (trout) fishing I could be ready in a few minutes—and not leave anything behind. The same would apply for my golf equipment and golf bag.

- Contracts, budgets, and other serious stuff: Many people are amazed at my "good memory." The truth is my memory is as good or as bad as anyone else's. However, I do the following: I do a summary (or an executive summary if you wish) of the important provisions of for instance a contract. These would normally include dates, amounts, escalation clauses, notice provisions, etc.

An example of such a summary could be: You rent an apartment to someone. I would typically give a short description of the apartment, followed by the important particulars of the contract: Sea and Stay, 23 Maxwell Street. Rent $6000 per month, payable first of each month. Escalation 10 percent per annum on 1 March. Tenant JH Smith. Letting agent. Notice period one calendar month.

My cell phone has the facility and memory capacity, so that I can offload this summary onto my phone. Whenever I have to wait at an airport or at the doctor's consulting rooms or for my wife to get dressed, I browse through these notes. It works especially well with complex contracts.

I do the same with a summary of the salient figures of a budget or financial statements. This would include turnover figures, stock levels, biggest expense figures, profits, net asset value, etc. I can assure you this method works, and it works because of the repetition of seeing these notes or figures at various (regular) intervals.

Do the same with investments. Note the yield, maturity dates, etc. When you read the note on investments, think about alternative investments, better yields, or more security for your investment. Keep your memory and brain busy.

- To do lists: I make lists of what I have to do before I go away or before a specific occasion, especially when I am pressed for time and am under a lot of work pressure. You could even use a standard list. My standard list for going abroad would for example look like this:

- Air tickets

- Identity document

- Drivers license (or international drivers license)

- Passport

- Chronic medications and a copy of the prescription

- Credit card and other money

- Extra pair of glasses (reading glasses). On one of my overseas trips my reading glasses got broken. It was really a struggle. If you do not have an extra pair of prescription reading glasses you can buy cheap nonprescription reading glasses at a pharmacy.

- Travel insurance and/or my medical aid card.

- Shopping lists: How many times have you not returned from the shops, only to remember (or being reminded) that you have not bought this or that. I make a list of things that I should buy. It works for me. This enables me to do my purchases reasonably quickly. It also helps me not to buy a lot of stuff I did not intend buying.

- Names: How many times have you been introduced to a person and to your embarrassment have forgotten the name after only a few moments? The secret is to use the name as many times as possible in the first minutes after you have met that person. Do not just say, "Pleased to meet you." Rather say, "Please to meet you, John," or "Pleased to meet you, Mr. Smith." Try to use the name and surname at least ten times in the first minutes after you have met the person, and you will be surprised how much better you remember the name.

Apart from the principle of repetition explained above, ask the person where he comes from, whether he is related to so and so, and what his favorite sport is. Anything to establish an association. If his surname is Black, you could see a huge container of black paint being emptied on his head. Remember that the color was black and not green. However, beware not to call him Mr. Green when you meet him again. Association is a powerful tool to use.

Lastly but very importantly, the moment you have a chance (and assuming it is important to you) enter his name into the contact list of your cell phone. If this person is accompanied by a partner, record the partner's name as well. If you meet this person again and have forgotten his name, the worst that can happen to you as that you could very discreetly look at your contact list.

• Passwords: What a nightmare to remember all the passwords you are using every day. You need a password to go into your bank account, to withdraw money from an automated teller machine, to get in and out of your estate, your alarm system at home or at the office, and to get in and out of the office and the parking garage. And if these are not enough, there are more passwords that you have to remember. I try to use the same password where possible. I also have different lists of passwords on my cell phone at different locations. From time to time I go through these passwords to ensure that I still remember them.

• My Action Book: I firmly believe that the smallest pencil is better than the biggest memory. Write down everything immediately. Do not delay, so that you will not forget to make an entry in your Action Book. Your Action Book is a reminder to act. Entries in my Action Book may look as follows:

1 September 2010: $100 000 invested with Bank A on a fixed deposit of 5 percent per annum. Maturity date 31 August 2011. (Also, immediately record 31 August 2011 (or earlier) to action this investment after maturity.)

2 September 2010: Joan borrowed *Gone with the Wind*. Will return it after the holidays in October.

3 September 2010: I agreed to help the bowling club with strategic planning. Call Henry Bruwer 082 55 1012 7 for the final arrangements. (Remember to record dates.)

Read through you Action Book every week at a fixed time. Take action where you have to. When I was doing my compulsory military service, I was in the engineering corps. Their motto was: What is possible, we do immediately—the impossible takes a little longer!

By simply following the guidelines above, everyone will be amazed on how much better your memory is and that you get things done. This is good news. Yes, you can do something about your memory. It's easy, it's fun, it costs you nothing extra, and most important of all—it works!

In the next chapter we discuss practical and fun ways to exercise your brain. Your brain needs to be exercised on a regular basis. If you do it, you will be surprised at the results.

A poor memory can have a very negative effect on the quality of your life. Do not spend hours and hours of your valuable life to look for your stuff. Do not accept a poor memory as a given. Don't forget to do something about your memory. Do it now!

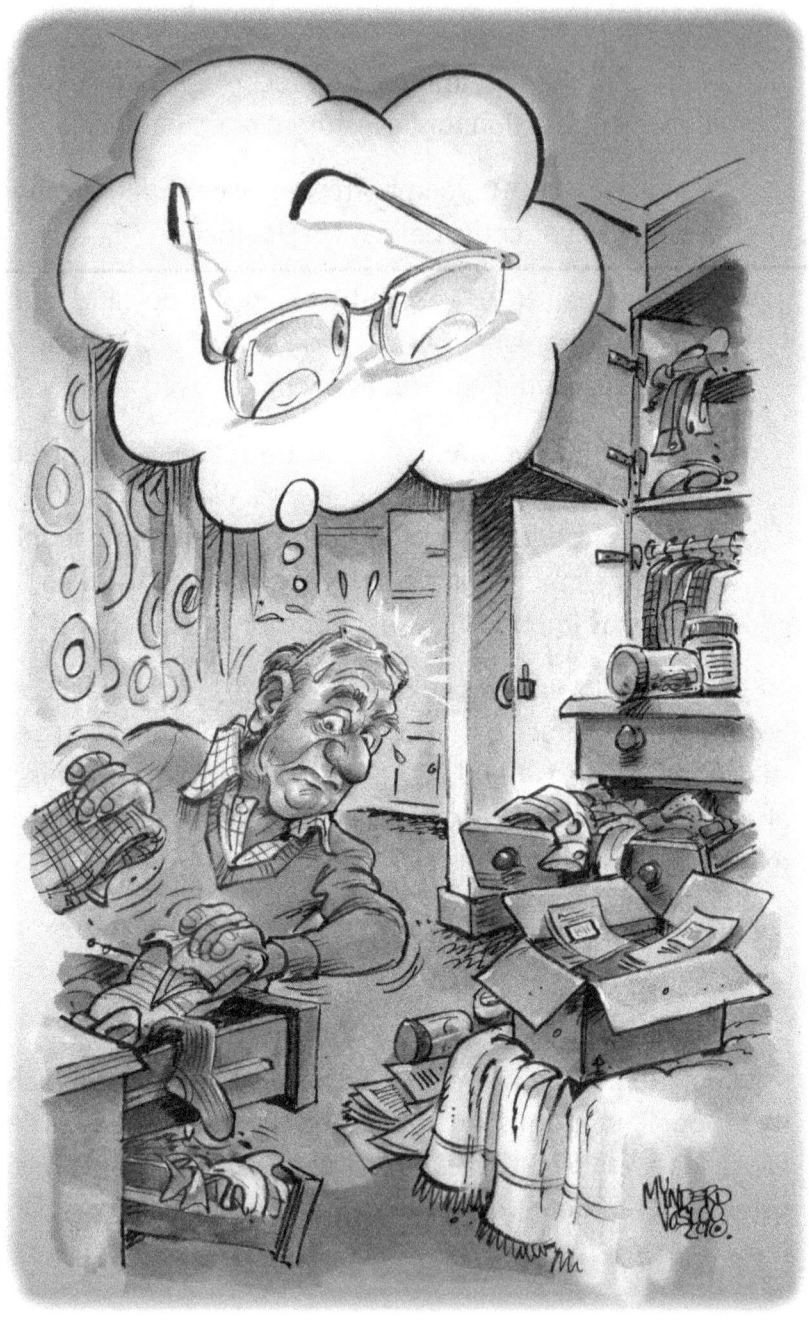

CHAPTER 4

EXERCISE THAT BRAIN

To keep our bodies in a healthy condition, we have to exercise regularly and correctly. The saying use it or lose it is very appropriate and very true. The very same principle applies to our brain. We must exercise that brain! It must be done regularly. It must be done on a daily basis. To exercise your brain is as important as exercising you body. Every day (yes, I mean *every* day) your brain must be exposed to something that is complex, difficult to understand, and hopefully sometimes forces your brain to really stretch itself to get a grip on the issue. For me it works well if I tackle something that is totally removed from my own (so-called) field of expertise. Do what works best for you. It is different for everyone. Here is an opportunity to fill your hours with something extraordinary and exciting. Come out of your comfort zone and start doing these brain exercises!

How do you exercise your brain daily? There are many practical and simple ways to do it.

When you attend a service in church:

- Try to repeat the essence of the sermon. What was it all about?

29

- What is the real message that was conveyed? How would you apply it in practice?

- When you sing during the service, the words of the song are sometimes projected electronically on the electronic board. Look at the sentence that you are singing, memorize the words quickly, then look away and sing the rest of the sentence without looking at the words again.

- Do the same when you sing from a hymnal. Later you can try to do two lines (sentences) of the song instead of only one. Yes, sometimes you might sing a slightly different word, but you will be amazed how effective this exercise is.

- When you need to read something out loud: As you read, read the rest of the sentence, quickly memorize the words, and complete the sentence without looking at the words again. When you look up from the book you are reading from and complete the sentence, it seems that you are so well prepared that you almost know it by heart. A bit of practice without an audience will give you a lot of confidence. Looking up from the book you are reading from and looking at the audience tend to help to hold the attention of the audience better.

When you attend a music concert, try to remember the names of the performing artists, what music they performed, and the names of the composer(s) of the music. Before the concert, search the Internet and read about the artist and also about the music and the composer. Make a point to discuss this information with a friend and share interesting facts with them. It is very informative and fun.

Fill out a SUDOKU every day. SUDOKU is a challenge to fill in the grid so that every row, every column, and every 3X3 grid contains the numerals one through nine with no repeats. This game is published in about every newspaper and magazine and on numerous Web sites. There are also different levels of difficulty. Once you have mastered a specific level, move on to the next level. SUDOKU is a good exercise for the brain. If you feel you have mastered the highest level, why not set up your own SUDOKU?

Do a crossword puzzle. Many people do not like to complete crossword puzzles. It remains a fun way to keep up your knowledge of a language and of synonyms, and it makes you think. Keep record on how you fared and try to improve on your previous best attempt.

Play a game that forces you to think and to concentrate, for example, to remember which cards have been played. Yes, I know sometimes it is nice just to play a game the result of which depends about 100 percent on the cards you have been dealt with. Even use a game of cards to exercise your brain. The challenge is to get the best possible result with whatever hand you are dealt with

Apart from card games, there are several other types of games you can play. It's fun and good exercise for your brain. I will mention three of those games, but there are many others.

One minute: its fun and a very good test for your general knowledge. When you determine a specific field where you lack the general knowledge, why not make a special effort to gain that knowledge! With the explosion of information on the Internet, it is easy and fun. Make up teams to play against each other.

Tri-ominos: This is a game that forces you to concentrate. Even when you are not playing, you have to look for opportunities to play when it is your turn.

Trivial Pursuit: This game probably needs no introduction. It deals with various fields of knowledge and a challenge for your general knowledge ranging from pop music to science.

Read the newspaper or specific articles in a scientific or economic journal. See if you can remember what the essence of the article is and if you can convey this to a friend. Sometimes you may think you understand something you read until you have to explain it to somebody else. Comment on reports in the magazine or newspaper and give your opinion, if this is your scene. Again there is a wealth of information about virtually any topic under the sun in libraries and on the Internet. Do not be afraid to use it!

If you are in any position to practice your hobby, do it. I know a number of senior citizens who do beautiful handiwork. The eye-hand coordination will do you the world of good. Do not just buy a design you want to use for embroidery or woodcarving—do the design yourself!

Do not tell me that the rheumatism in your hands is so bad that you cannot practice your hobby. Read the chapter on age is no excuse again. When this happened to Grandma Moses and she was unable to carry on with her embroidery, she started painting and became a world famous American folk artist.

If your hobby is photography, you can find out about all the electronic gadgets you can think off to improve your techniques. By effectively using these digital gadgets your videos and pictures can almost be professional quality. This also enables you to do incredible photo series with beautiful music. You can turn those old slides and films into digital recordings or videos. Even better, get the equipment and do all the transitions to digital format yourself. The possibilities are endless. Just do something!

However, you cannot do all the above and a host of other interesting things unless you are reasonably comfortable to use your computer. There are many user-friendly programs that make it relatively easy to do very interesting things. The Internet provides access to information on about every subject on this planet. It does not matter what your interests are—you will find information on that subject on the Internet. Do not be afraid to use the Internet to its fullest extent. Use the Internet—it is fun and very informative.

If you would like to play chess and you have nobody to play against, it is also not a problem. You can play against the computer. There are numerous programs to accommodate you. You can also choose what level of difficulty you would like to tackle. Keep a record and try to improve on the results.

If you cannot play chess, why do you not start learning? Again there are many programs on the Internet available to teach you how to play chess. You are never too old to learn.

The key is, do something! Whatever it is you want to do! Do not just sit in the sitting room or in front of the television set and wait for death to come!

When last did you learn a poem by heart? What about a few paragraphs or two of beautiful prose? You can still do it!

Are you a member of a book club (where members discuss different books they read or new publications on the market). If you are not a member, why do you not join a book club? If there is no book club and you would have liked to be a member of such a club, why don't you establish one? Do not just be an onlooker, but take an active part. Offer to do a book review. Get interesting facts about that book and its author from the Internet. The secret is preparation. Be well prepared and talk about the new book release with confidence. You will have the confidence if you are well prepared.

Do the same if you belong to a Bible study group. Volunteer to present the discussion. Again prepare properly. There are a magnitude of reference books and bewildering loads of information on the Internet. Go the extra mile and present something you can really be proud off. You'll be astonished what it does to your confidence and your self-image. Let the adrenalin flow. Above all—enjoy it.

There is absolutely no excuse why you have to be a "sleeping" member (literally and figuratively) of any group you belong to.

I usually do calculations and additions on the computer. To exercise the brain, I sometimes do it without using any tools and just check my answers with the computer. I like to add up the figures of the stuff I buy at a supermarket as I put them into the trolley (in round figures) and then check my calculations against the cashier's total at the till. I do this for the fun of it. So why don't you try it the next time you go shopping? It is a fun game to play.

If you are one of the fortunate ones who can also play a musical instrument, do not stop doing it, especially if you read music notes. It is not only a great general therapy, but also very good exercise in hand-eye-brain coordination.

Now here is something I like to do. When you enter any room, note how many windows and doors there are in the room. Note the furniture, the paintings, and where and how these are arranged in the room. After you have left and when you have a chance try to put the detail of that room on paper. If possible, go back to that room and compare what you did from memory to the real situation. Do this exercise for a number of times. You will be astonished how your ability to observe will improve over a period of time. Naturally your amazing memory should impress many of your friends.

I am sure you will be able to invent many more and more interesting brain exercises. The secret is to use that brain! What is true about the muscles of your body is equally true of your brain: Use it or lose it!

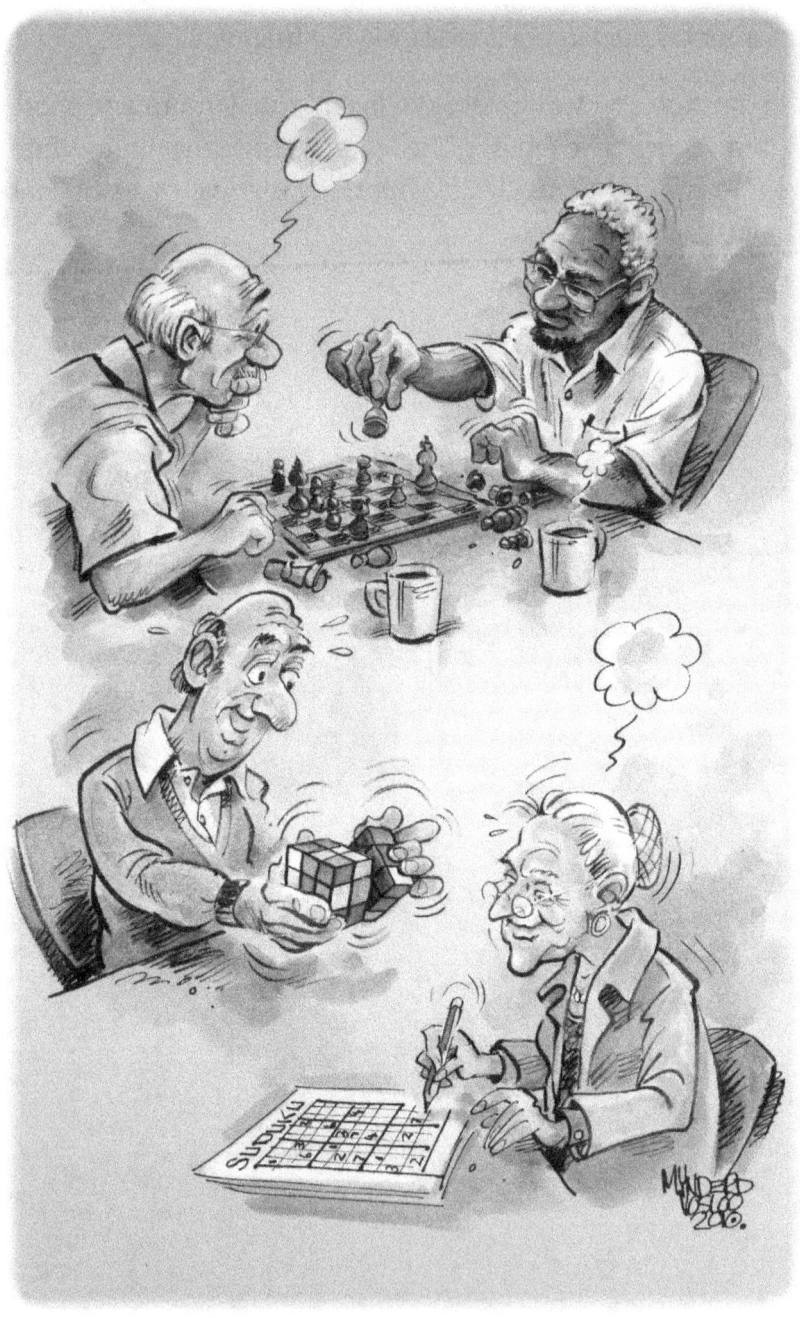

CHAPTER 5

AND NOW THOSE PILLS

Many senior people are on medication of some sort. Perhaps a bigger number of us are on chronic medication. A serious problem amongst senior people is that they do not take important prescribed medicine regularly. In many other instances older people are taking excessive medication because they simply cannot remember whether they have already taken their medicine.

Can any of you honestly say that you are taking your pills strictly according to the medical practitioner's prescription? It may also happen that you just cannot remember whether you have taken your pills and just for safety sake take the full doses again. In this way you can easily take too few pills (underdosage) or too many pills (overdosage). Both overdosage and underdosage can be dangerous for your health and should be avoided at all times.

There are very good reasons why medication should be taken as prescribed. Huge amounts of money are spent on research and development of medicine. Medical practitioners and pharmacists study many years to enable them to prescribe the right quantities that we should take for the benefit of our health. The least we can do is to ensure that we take the medication as prescribed.

The good news is that there is a whole range of practical and inexpensive methods you can use to ensure you take your medications properly.

Probably the easiest way is to buy an inexpensive pillbox that is able to hold your pills for each day of the week. Each little compartment is clearly marked for the specific day of the week. These pillboxes are also made of plastic and can be bought at most pharmacies or pharmaceutical outlets. It is normally inexpensive. The seven-day pillboxes are divided into seven sections or compartments and each section is meant for the pills for that specific day. The seven sections are usually marked for each day of the week, and some are further divided to provide for your morning, afternoon, and evening medications. At the beginning of the week, you could fill up the entire pillbox for everyday of the week. You can now easily see whether you have taken your medication by simply look-ing at the section for that day. In the case of chronic medica-tion, you can see in advance whether you must get your new prescription for your chronic medication.

By using this pillbox you no longer need to depend on your weakening memory to ensure that you take your medication regularly and correctly.

If you no longer see properly, or are unsure of the dosages, always ask someone else to help you.

This pillbox is very convenient if you want to go away for a weekend or on holiday. Just ensure that you have enough pills for the number of days you will be away. Then you simply pack your pillbox and off you go.

Remember to always have your pillbox as part of your hand baggage when you are traveling by air. In case your other luggage gets lost, you have your chronic (or other) medicine with you. By following these very basic guidelines you not only ensure that you do not forget your medicine at home, but you also ensure that you have your medicine with you even if your other luggage gets lost.

As one might expect, there are quite many variations and different types of pillboxes. Some pillboxes can even take a month's medication. There are more expensive electronic pillboxes with an alarm to remind you to take your pills. Use the one that works for you and make it part of your daily life.

If you do not have a pillbox, you can still take the correct medication. If you have to take more than one kind of pill, do the following: Take every pill from the container, put them together, and take all the pills at once. After I have taken a pill from its container, I put that bottle and box to one side, so I know I have taken those pills out already. Take your pills at the same time every day, such as after meals. By doing this it becomes a habit and you tend not to forget to take your pills.

Unfortunately, we sometimes get medication in other forms than pills, like eye drops or medicines in liquid form. I am not aware of a simple device that solves the taking of this type of medication as easily as a pillbox. For this type of medicine, it is probably most practical to set an alarm to remind you to take your medication. The alarm on your watch or cell phone could be ideal for this. Most of the electronic alarms can be set to go off every day at a specific time. One can even change the alarm's tone to remind you to take the medication.

I am also aware that you can get SMS messages on your mobile phone to remind you to take your medication. It is not widely used, and I do not know how expensive and practical it is.

It does not matter which method you use to ensure that you take your medicine correctly and regularly. Get a method that works for you.

It is very important that you refrain from taking just any pill, especially those recommended by your hairdresser or the pills recommended by your golf partners. Use only the pills prescribed by a registered medical practitioner. Before taking any other pills, ask your medical practitioner or your qualified pharmacist for their expert opinion. Your medical practitioner or pharmacist will ensure it does not clash with any of your other medication and that it is in your interest to use those pills.

There is another form of overdoses that can be very dangerous to your health. What I am referring to is not following the instructions on the leaflet (pamphlet) that is packed with the medication to the letter. You can buy a medicine over the counter for the symptomatic relief of the common cold and influenza, sinusitis, hay fever, and postnasal drip (amongst others). On this leaflet there is also a warning: "Do not use continuously for more than ten days without consulting your doctor as severe liver damage may be caused." You get older people who simply don't read these leaflets and in any case totally ignore this very important warning!

Now those "wonder" pills and cures. These are the pills that are guaranteed (whatever "guaranteed" means) to make you younger, to lose many kilograms and get your weight under control, to take away all those wrinkles, to stimulate hair growth, to increase your virility, and many, many other impossibilities. Beware, beware, and beware! Normally these spell problems. See the danger lights flickering. If, despite this warning, you are convinced you want to use it, first consult your medical practitioner or your qualified pharmacist. I shall be surprised if they are happy for you to use these "medications."

I read about a lady who went into a cosmetics shop to buy a new antiageing face cream which, according to the advert is "guaranteed" to make the years drop off. Following the instructions carefully she religiously applies just the right amount twice a day and waits expectantly for the results.

After a few weeks, she decides that it's time to see if her husband has noticed any difference. One evening before bed she plucks up the courage to ask him. "Darling, tell me the truth, what age would you say I am?"

Looking her up and down her husband replies, "Well, Susan, judging from your skin—twenty, your hair—eighteen, and your figure—twenty-five." His wife gushed, "Oh, you flatterer!" She kissed him and turned to leave. "Hey, wait a minute," he called. "I haven't added them up yet."[3]

Back to serious issues: Many of these wonder cures are not registered medication. Please remember that large pharmaceutical companies spend billions of dollars in research and development for new medication. It takes years of testing and further development before new medication is registered.

Recently in the newspapers in South Africa and on the television channels, there was much discussion about all kinds of vitamins and mineral supplements that people take. You might also be aware that these supplements are quite expensive. The conclusion reached by the majority of authors and

---

3 Shelly Klein, *The Little Book of Senior Moments* (London: Michael O'Hara Books, 2008), 60.

presenters of programs was that most of these supplements make little or no contribution to people's general health.

The guideline is simple: Ask your medical practitioner or at least your pharmacists whether it is necessary for you to take such supplements. Use the money you save on all kinds of supplements (that are not prescribed by your medical practitioner) for other good things in life.

It is not very clever to abuse your body. You only have one body, and this body has to last you until you die. Look after this body very well. Follow a conservative policy regarding your health. Your medical practitioner did not study medicine for all those years just for the fun of it. Your medical professional is in the best position to advise you properly on all medical matters.

Regular and comprehensive medical examinations are of utmost importance. You must under no circumstances decide to skip it because you are feeling well. If health problems are diagnosed in time, even if these problems are serious, your chances of surviving are so much better. Men must especially be vigilant for prostate problems, and men and women for various cancers and other diseases. You always have a better chance of recovery (and survival) if a problem is discovered and properly treated in time.

A regular visit to the dentist is equally important. If you do not have your natural teeth, the health of your gums and your overall oral hygiene is very important. Apart from other disorders, your gums could be the cause of bad breath.

To summarize: It is of the utmost importance to take prescribed medication correctly and regularly. Go to a proper registered medical practitioner for your health problems and get the right medicine. Be very cautious about all these wonder cures and do not use them unless prescribed by your medical practitioner. Go for regular medical checkups and do not forget oral hygiene.

Prevention is better than cure, especially when it comes to health matters. If you can stay reasonably healthy, it will greatly contribute to a quality lifestyle.

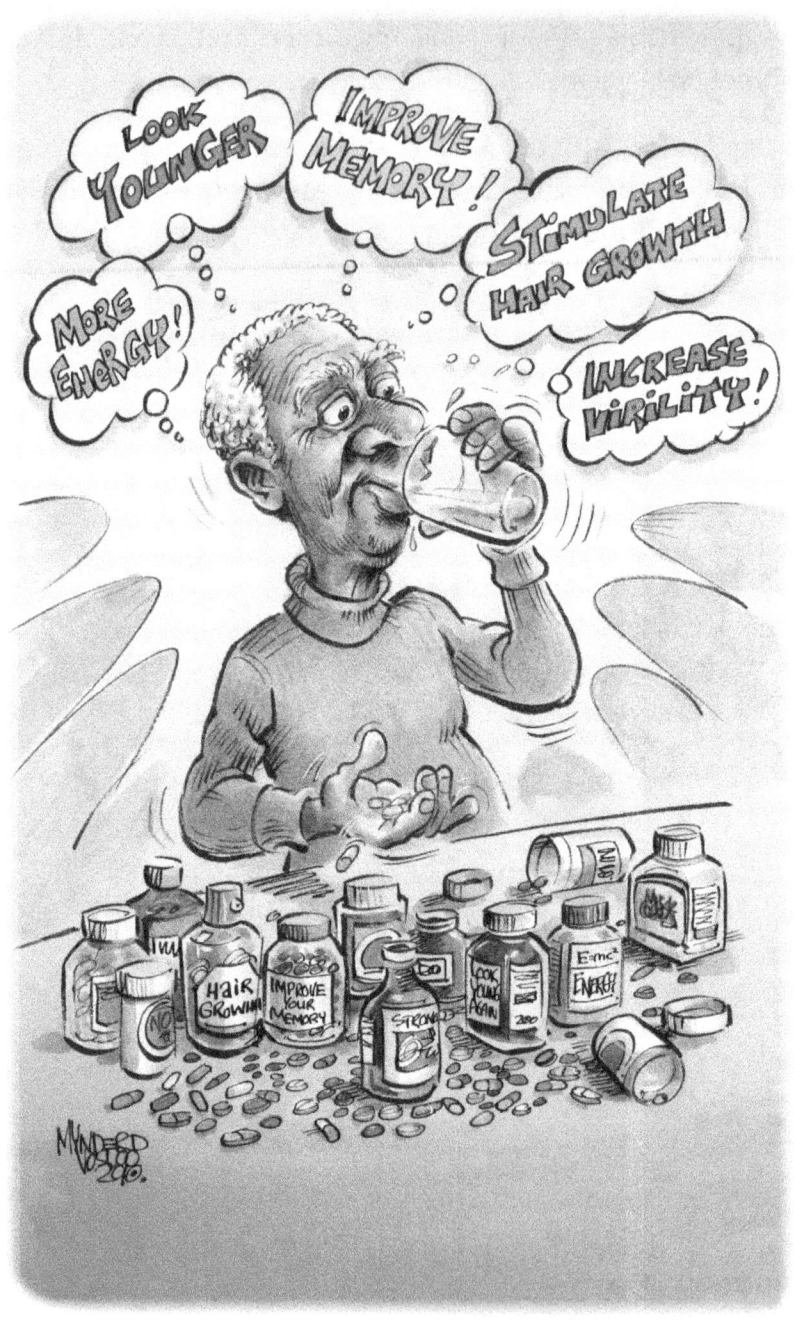

CHAPTER 6

MONEY MATTERS

Money matters? Yes, it matters! Let's talk about money in simple terms.

We read in financial magazines that most people who retire did not make adequate provision for their retirement. This can prove to really become a big headache for many of our fellow senior citizens. The question inevitably is: Do I have enough money to enable me to lead (or maintain) a quality lifestyle until I die?

Another problem is that we do not know how long our lives will be. If we knew how old we are going to get, it would have been very easy to calculate how much money we need. The arithmetic is quite simple. Take the total capital/investments you now have, taking into account what the proceeds on your capital/investments will be, and determine what the balance of your total estate should be at the time of your death. All you have to do now is to divide the total amount available by the numbers of years to death. This is what you have available to spend every year—and voilà, go for the jackpot.

Unfortunately it is not that simple. There are too many unknown factors that will affect this calculation. Even the so-called experts struggle to come up with a reasonable answer.

- How long you're going to live

- What will your health be like

- What will the returns/proceeds on your capital/ investments going to be

- What about direct and indirect taxes on revenue and capital income/gains

- What are the prospects for capital growth

- What is the role that inflation will play and what is the expected impact of inflation on your planning

- How much of your capital should still be available at the end of your lifetime (either to cover all the costs on death or how much your heirs should inherit)

The above are just some of the uncertainties that could substantially influence your capital, income, and expenses. It is under these uncertainties that we have to plan for our old age as best as we can. This is indeed a challenge.

There are two ways to respond to this challenge. The first is to get so overwhelmed by these uncertainties that you throw in the towel and do no planning at all. The second and positive approach is to gather all available and relevant information and in (or with) the light you have at that stage, do your financial planning to the best of your ability. From this it follows that this is not a once off exercise. You have to continuously address these issues as more current information becomes available and circumstances change.

The point is you must plan for your old age. Even more so if you think you did not make adequate provision. In that case it is even more important to do forward planning. Fortunately there are experts to help you. It's highly unlikely that you (or the experts) will forecast the financial markets correctly. Nobody can, but at least give it your best effort.

The majority of my fellow senior citizens are no longer economically active. This means that these people are not in a position to increase their capital. They will have to survive on their capital already accumulated up to their retirement date and live off the proceeds of their capital. The proceeds on the capital invested could be supplemented by annuity income and pension income. I refer to the total of the proceeds of the capital and any other income as the total income of a person. The question then is whether your total income is sufficient to support your present lifestyle.

The dilemma that we face is that our capital amount is fixed. The capital is fixed in the sense that we are unable to increase our capital (and therefore the proceeds on it) if our cost of living increases. The proceeds on our capital are further subject to fluctuations of interest rates and the declaration of dividends by a board of directors and we have practically no say in the dividend policy of a big company.

In our planning we have to take a very critical look at our cost of living. In many instances it can be reduced or consolidated.

I divide my living expenses into three categories:

- Must have (such as food, clothing, taxes, and medical provisions)

- Should have (to enable me to live a reasonable quality life such as a good residence, quality furniture, motor vehicle, etc)

- Great to have (holiday home, farm, recreation vehicles, overseas travel, safari, etc.)

If my living expenses are more than my total income, I know immediately where to cut expenses. I go back to my "great to have" category and determine what I can do without.

Another possibility to solve this problem is to determine whether you can increase your total income. It may be that you can convert existing investments with low returns to investments with higher returns. Quite recently I discussed this possibility with my broker, and it was no surprise to me that we could switch the investment to companies with a higher dividend yield without increasing risk. One could also switch to an investment to get increased after tax returns. For example: Presently in South Africa normal dividends are not taxed. The return you receive is therefore a return after tax. There are many possibilities and you can discuss all the possibilities with financial experts. However, keep the following guidelines in mind:

- Yield and risk usually go hand in hand. The greater the yield, the greater the risk.

  If you have to move your investments between different funds, there could be costs involved. Always determine what the total cost is to make or change any investment.

- Never invest in an enterprise, scheme, or structure you do not fully understand. It must be very clear to you what happens to the monies you invest and how the income will be generated.

  An investment too good to be true is too good to be true. Beware and do not touch it!

- Invest only in and through accredited and reputable (normally well known) financial institutions

- If you have to err, err on the conservative side. Rather be safe than sorry.

Another important issue we have to consider is using your capital (albeit a small part) for your day-to-day living expenses (consumption of capital). Say that you have cut your cost of living and have increased your total income within the above guidelines, but you are still unable to finance your cost of living. You have therefore to supplement this shortfall with something else. You are unable to cut further on your living expenses and you are unable to increase the return on your investments. You may now decide to make up the shortfall by using part of your capital to do this. However, if you do this, you will be "eating" into your capital, and your capital will become smaller and smaller. At the age of sixty and with a relative long life expectancy, I shall be reluctant to do this. At the age of say eighty years, it is easier to take the decision to use part of your capital. This will result in a smaller capital and estate on your death. For many this is not really a problem!

As your capital gets smaller, the return on your capital will be reduced proportionately. This in turn may force you to use a bigger portion of your capital. This may further decrease the return on your capital.

If you have to make the decision to use part of your capital to finance your cost of living, you should at least follow the following guideline: Select the asset with the lowest returns and the asset with the poorest prospects for capital growth. You will also have taken the market conditions into account and whether the market of that particular asset is a buyers market or a sellers market. Discuss this with an expert before you make your decision.

We must continually try to at least maintain our total income. This is our first goal. This means that we strive to (at least) keep the total income on the same income levels.

Our second goal is to increase our total income and improve the return on our capital. This is not easy, but nobody said it is going to be.

How can you maintain and even improve your total income? Here are three guidelines to help you to achieve this.

- Try to avoid using part of your capital for your cost of living. If you do this your capital gets smaller and smaller, and so does you return on investment.

- Should your total income exceed the amount needed for your living expenses, invest this surplus properly. By doing this you increase the amount of your investments and can hopefully increase your total income.

- If the return on your investments can beat inflation, you are well on your way to achieve this.

To make investments that beat inflation is easier said than done. Investment advisers sometimes claim that the investment they recommend can easily beat inflation. The next time somebody tells you that, let that person explain exactly how the proposed investment will beat inflation.

To be able to judge whether an investment will beat inflation, we have to know what the practical effects of inflation on our money matters are.

What is inflation?

There are many definitions for inflation, but for purposes of this book we shall keep it as simple as possible. Inflation is the continual rise in the prices of goods and services with the result that the buying power of your currency gets smaller all the time. In practical terms it means that for the same amount of money, you can buy less goods and services. Immediately it is clear that people with a fixed total income, will be effected by inflation—sometimes even seriously affected. It is thus clear that inflation has a major impact on financial planning for your old age. It has indeed!

Let us illustrate this with an example:

You have made an investment (like a fixed deposit). On this investment you receive a fixed income after tax of $100,000 per annum. Suppose your total living expenses are $100,000 per annum. In year one, there is no problem. You can (in year one) finance your living expenses of $100,000 per annum from the proceeds of $100,000 (after tax) from your fixed investment.

Suppose the inflation rate is 6 percent. This means that the price of the goods and services will increase by 6 percent (or put in other words, the buying power of your money has been eroded (reduced) by 6 percent). Goods and services that previously cost $100,000, now cost $106,000 ($100,000, plus 6 percent of $100,000). The problem is that the return on your fixed investment after tax did not change and is still $100,000 after tax. This means you now have a deficit of $6,000 to maintain the same standard of living (or to buy the same goods and services you bought the previous year). If you want to be in the same position you were in year one, you are now faced with three choices:

Choice 1: Cut back on your living expenses (buy fewer goods and services) to the amount of $6,000.

Choice 2: Increase your total income after tax with $6,000 and keep your living expenses at the same level.

Choice 3: Do both: cut back on your living expenses and increase your total income to the point where you can again buy the goods and services you could afford in year one.

Many of us older people do not have the luxury of these choices. One tends to be reluctant to cut down on your cost of living. Sometimes, and depending on the market, it is very difficult to maintain your total income, and almost impossible to increase your total income.

What happens if you cannot increase your total income and cannot reduce your living expenses?

In this unfortunate situation you might have no choice but to use part of your capital (investments) to fund your cost of living. You can guess what happens next. Because your investments (capital) get smaller and smaller, the return on your investments (and your total income) gets smaller and smaller. Because your total income is smaller and prices are still rising (because of inflation), you have to use more of your capital (investments) to supplement the deficit. This could become a vicious circle with you caught up in the middle of it.

From the example above it is clear that not only will inflation influence your total income but will also erode the buying power of your investments (capital). In a world of year-on-year inflation, the buying power of your total income and the buying power of your capital (investments) will simply become smaller, and you will buy less with the same amount of money.

Inflation has thus a serious impact on the capital you invested and the proceeds of that capital. Here are more practical examples of the influence of inflation:

Suppose you have invested an amount of $100,000 as a fixed deposit at an interest rate of 5 percent after tax. You do not need the interest to cover your cost of living. Suppose the inflation rate is 5 percent and remains at 5 percent. At the end of year one, you reinvest the interest after tax (5 percent of $100,000 = $5,000) under the same conditions. Your total investment is $100,000 plus $5,000 = $105,000. Your interest after tax on $105,000 is now $5,250. If you again reinvest the interest after tax the $,250, your investment will keep pace with inflation. This means that the purchasing power of your fixed deposit plus the reinvested interest after tax, remained intact.

Please note that in the above example the investment could only keep up with inflation because you were in a position to reinvest the interest after tax. If you had to use the interest as part of your cost of living, the purchase power of your $100,000 investment would simply be reduced by the rate of inflation.

Here is another example: We use the same numbers as in the example directly above but a different type of asset. Suppose you have a fixed property with a market value of $100,000 that you rent out for 5 percent after tax. The inflation rate is 5 percent and stays at 5 percent. Let us assume that the prices of properties increase by the same rate as inflation. The lease agreement provides that the escalation in rent will be calculated, so that the annual rent also increases with the inflation rate. In this example, your investment (fixed property) kept pace with inflation. This is so because the market value of the property rose with the same rate as the inflation rate. What's more, your return on this investment also kept pace with inflation. Even if you use your rental income as part of your cost of living (and not reinvest the rental income) your investment is not effected by inflation. This is so as we have assumed in our example that the prices of property will increase at the same rate as inflation.

If you have a situation where you have to pay capital gains tax, you have to take this tax into account when realizing the property.

What you are looking for is an investment that appreciates with at least the rate of inflation, and a return on investment that increases year on year with at least the rate of inflation. This would be the ideal inflation-resistant investment.

Next time someone wants to sell you an inflation-resistant investment, you know what questions to ask and how to do your sums.

During the recent worldwide recession, the value of investments decreased considerably. Particularly listed shares were affected severely. Although many quality shares recovered very well, it is highly unlikely that share prices in the shorter-to-medium term will get to the same level as the prices before the recession. The market for fixed property was also affected and eventually property prices stabilized on levels that are lower than those before the worldwide recession. This means that with respect to both fixed property and listed shares, one can talk about a permanent decline in the value of these investments. How would a permanent decline in the value of investments affect the older people?

It is well to remember that even when there is a permanent decline in the value of an asset, the return on such an asset need not necessarily to decline. It is possible that the value of fixed property is reduced, but that the rental income of that fixed property will remain the same or could even increase. This is so because the rental income is based on the rent agreement and the rent agreement can even make provision for an escalation of rent. If you do not need to sell the property for some or other reason, and are looking at the fixed property as a long-term investment, the decrease in the value of the property is not a problem. The market value of the property will normally rise again as the economic environment changes to sustained growth.

It goes without saying that if you have to realize the asset during a period of falling prices, the loss is realized and the total value of your capital will be reduced.

For the sake of completeness, I would just like to mention that there might be other assets on which you do not receive a return as such. A good example of this type of asset is a holiday home. Even if you do not rent the holiday home to outsiders, you can regard the amount what you would have paid for holiday accommodation, as the return on this investment. If the holiday home was bought or built at a good price, the seemingly ever-rising market for some holiday homes could go a long way to offset inflation.

Due to excellent health care and also a healthy lifestyle, we tend to live longer and reach a higher age. Life expectancy tables verify this fact. Your chance to live longer than the general expectation a few decades ago is excellent. It's probably good news. The bad news is you will need more money to be able to live or to maintain your standard of living for a longer period of time that you initially planned. It is therefore of the utmost importance to preserve your capital (investments), as well as you can (or is allowed to by inflation and other market conditions).

The guideline is: Preserve your capital (investments), and if at all possible, increase it.

This brings us back to another practical problem. It gets quite emotional. The reasoning goes, more or less like this: Our children are in need of their inheritance now. Why wait until the death of the surviving spouse before they can get their inheritance or part thereof? If our heirs could get their inheritance now it will give them a tremendous financial boost. Of course it is true, but also keep in mind what is written above on the havoc inflation can play on your investments and total income.

If you have to decide whether or not to give your heirs part of their inheritance, there are easy guidelines to apply in these circumstances. Your first financial objective is to ensure that you are not a financial burden on your children or on the state. How do you calculate that? The answer is to calculate your surplus capital. For this purpose surplus capital is the capital remaining after you have calculated the capital (investments) you need to invest to lead and maintain a quality life until you die. For this purpose, you have to take into account the effect of inflation on your calculations. Even if you think you can do this sum yourself, get an expert to check your calculations. If the answer is that you do have surplus capital, you can distribute your surplus capital amongst your heirs.

Earlier we discussed the guideline: Preserve your capital (investments), and if at all possible, increase it. This is easier said than done. Actually it is in our efforts to preserve our capital and increase our total income that we can easily get lost in a minefield of misinformation. We have to be very wary of the many pitfalls in this area. Why? It seems that older people have become the target of all of the villains, tricksters and psychopaths of this world. There are too many sad stories where older people have literally lost everything and now live in the greatest of poverty.

How can you identify these impostors? The following is usually the fraudsters' methodology:

- The returns offered on the investments are much higher than the returns of recognized reputable financial institutions.

- Presenter is vague when asked why the yield is so much higher than other "normal" investments. This vagueness is supplemented by mentioning financial instruments you have never heard off.

- You do not understand completely what you are offered, but the crook is so convincing that you feel comfortable. In many instances these salespeople are very smooth talkers.

- You do not really understand the investment opportunity and think it is because of your lack of financial knowledge.

- The salesperson cannot give you names of other people who already have made millions because the information is highly confidential. Besides, you may not offer this to other people or talk to other people about this. This offer is only for you. Do not miss out on this once in a lifetime opportunity.

- If you ask for time to study the matter properly or to discuss it with an expert, the answer normally is that because of this or the other reason, there is no further time to waste. If you do not immediately sign the investment form and pay over your money, you will miss this outstanding and secure investment opportunity.

- As a special favor just for you, these huge returns can be invested in a "tax haven" on your behalf. So, you pay no tax on these huge returns thus making the investment even more attractive. All you have to do is to pay over your money, sit back, and watch yourself getting richer and richer all the time.

If anyone would approach you with any of the above nonsense, do not even listen. Just hold on tightly to your money and run. Do not even give it a second thought. This is a scam. If you would invest with such a person, all you are going to achieve is to lose your money. This is guaranteed. Run!

What should you do?

- Use only approved and registered investment advisers. No, your hairdresser is not such an adviser.

- Invest only with reputable recognized financial institutions. Everyone knows who these institutions are. Avoid banks or other financial institutions that you have not heard of. Use only approved and known financial institutions, even though the returns on your investments might be lower.

- Forget about get-rich-quick money schemes; they really do not exist. This you should know at your age.

- Be conservative in your investment strategy. For us seniors a conservative strategy gives the best long-term results.

- Make sure you know exactly what the total cost of the investment is and what the investment adviser's total compensation is.

- Never invest in anything you do not fully understand. Remember that risk and return usually go hand in hand, and the higher the yield, the higher the risk. If a return on an investment is too good to be true, it is too good to be true.

- Do not be afraid to get good advice. Within reason, good advice is worth every cent you pay for it.

- Enter into investment management contracts with reputable managers. Ensure that you fully understand the cost and financial implications of the contract. Take into account your total cost of investment when calculating your effective return on your investments.

- I consider Warren Buffet's investment performance as one of the biggest successes ever. Warren Buffet does not invest in any financial scheme or company whose business he not properly understands. If Warren Buffet does not understand everything, why would you? Buffet also does not invest in a company if he is not convinced that the management of the company is efficient and trustworthy.

Again do not sign any contract or agreement until you really understand what you are signing. Ask questions until you get all the answers you need. If necessary, ask why certain clauses are in the contract and why there is not enough protection for you. Rather get the reputation that you do not put your signature to any document easily, than the other way round.

Some of the agreements for the provision of investment management services have a clause that the contract will be automatically renewed until cancelled by you. In many instances this also means an escalation of management costs. Do not accept this condition. Rather have a clause that stipulates you are able to evaluate the investment manager's performance and then decide whether you would want to renew the contract.

In my view the only effective way to evaluate the performance of an investment manager, is to monitor the real rate of return of your income and whether your capital has increased at a rate at least the same or higher than the inflation rate.

When it comes to returns on investments there are in reality two yields of interest. The first is the nominal rate of return. This is the rate that the bank will offer you on your investment. Let's say the interest rate is such that it gives 5 percent per year after tax. Let us assume that the inflation rate is 3 percent. This means that the real rate of return (or after inflation rate of return) on your investment is 2 percent (5 percent less 3 percent).

If you use the above example but we assume that the inflation rate now rises to 7 percent, the real return on investment will be minus 2 percent (7 percent minus 5 percent). This means that even if you reinvest the total after tax return (5 percent) the buying power of your investment will slowly be deteriorating.

So the real rate of return is the following:

- The return on investments
- Less: Management fees
- Less: Tax
- Less: Inflation
- = Real return on investments.

You also have to look at your real growth of investments (capital). Real growth of investments is

- The growth from the previous evaluation period, as reflected through share prices, property prices, etc.
- Less: Management fees
- Less: Calculated Capital Gains Tax

- Less: inflation

- = Real growth on investments

When you do the evaluation of the effectiveness of the management of your investments, you can use the following guidelines:

- What was the real return on your investments?

- What is the real growth of your investments (capital)

- How do these compare with the previous evaluation period and what are the explanations for any significant deviation?

- What is the investment strategy for the next period to achieve a real return on investments and real growth of the investments?

Some senior citizens enjoy a usufruct. A usufruct arose mostly in terms of a will when the surviving spouse is entitled to a usufruct for life. This means that the surviving spouse may use the return on an asset for life, but may not sell the asset. The usufruct could have arisen from a condition in the will that an asset (for example fixed property) belonging to the deceased should be sold, the selling price invested and that the surviving spouse would enjoy the returns of the investment for life. A usufruct could be an important asset, so treat it as such.

In everyday life one finds that there can be a lot of pressure on older people to sign off the usufruct because the children need to realize the asset because of their financial situation. Do not sign off this usufruct unless you have discussed this with an expert and you really understand the implications of signing off this usufruct. A usufruct should be replaced with another asset that provides the same privileges as the original

usufruct. Do not forget to bring into account the effect of inflation and tax in your calculations.

Certain annuities are paid out from the returns of a capital
sum to be invested on your behalf. You are allowed to annually choose what percentage of the total investment available
(between legally prescribed limits) you would like to receive
as a pension. Should the amount that you wish to receive be
more than the return on the investment, it means that part of
your pension is paid out of capital. This means that you have
to take into account that the amount of the capital invested
will become smaller and smaller (and hence the returns would
become smaller and smaller). If this continues, your monthly
pension will eventually be very small and eventually stop
altogether.

Remember to keep your income tax up to date. It is just not
worth it to get behind on your tax payments. Even if you deem
yourself to be a tax expert, get a tax expert to assist you. Tax
laws change every year, and you might not be up to date with
the newest legislation. On incorrect returns you might be pay-
ing excessive tax or pay penalties in the form of double taxa-
tion. On late tax payments you have to pay interest. Interest
payable to tax authorities is normally not tax deductable. All
these penalties and interest payable to the tax authorities are
simply a waste of money. Get a tax expert to assist you!

Never get involved in funny and suspicious schemes to avoid
tax—it does not work. In the long run it could result in additional taxes, penalties, interest payments, and even criminal
offences. That does not mean that you can do proper tax planning with the assistance of a reputable tax expert or a recognized tax consultant. There is no reason at all why you should
not do it. My advice is to do it properly.

Good advice for a friend might not be good advice for you. Each person's circumstances are unique. Get an expert to help you find the best solutions for your particular circumstances.

Please remember:

- If something is too good to be true, it is too good to be true. Do not touch such an "investment."

- Risk and yield go hand in hand: The higher the yield, the higher the risk. Be careful.

- Follow a conservative investment approach. Err on the conservative side.

- The time for taking risks is gone. You should have done that at a much younger age.

- The effective measurement for managing investments is real rate of return on investments and real growth of investments.

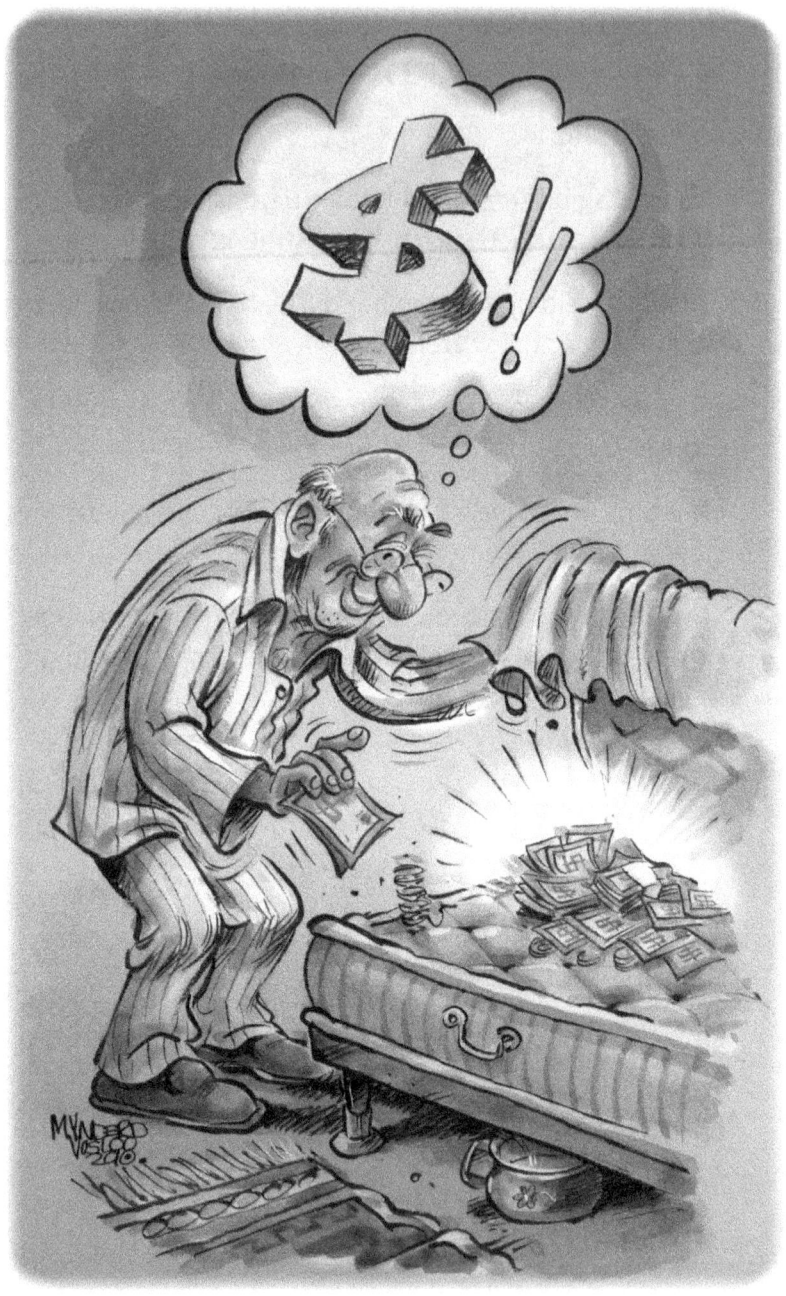

CHAPTER 7

YOUR LAST WILL

Remember that this is your last will. This means that this would be your last instructions that somebody (usually the executor of your estate) has to act on and carry out. This is a very important document and can be changed anytime before your death.

This is *your* last will not the last will of somebody else. Make sure that this document contains what you really want to happen with your assets after your death. It is your good right to bequeath your assets to whom and in what way you like. If you and your spouse have decided that you would bequeath your assets jointly, you should jointly agree on exactly how this will be done.

Make sure your will is written in plain and clear language that leaves no doubt to any reader of the will what exactly should happen on your death. Be very specific and do not be vague about any matter. If for instance you want to leave it to the discretion of your executor when to sell listed shares (depending on the market conditions), state it very clearly and for what period this discretion should be exercised.

Review your will regularly. Especially when the following happen:

- A divorce

- You remarry

- Worldwide recession

- When your financial position change substantially after buying or selling important assets

- If the political instability could affect future planning

- When your health deteriorates drastically

- A sharp increase in the inflation rate

You will be amazed how a person's circumstances could change in a short period of time. Review your will at least once a year. I review my will usually annually when I have to file my income tax returns.

Read your will carefully as if you are an outsider and ensure that all the terms and conditions are very clear and not ambiguous. When the executor of your will has to interpret your will, you will not be around to tell your executor what you actually meant. It goes without saying that you should avoid any Latin or legal terms that you do not fully understand. My advice is do not use that terminology at all. Again, use simple and clear language. If your will is drafted by somebody else, make sure that you tell this to that person.

Why am I so serious on why you should revise your will regularly? You will be amazed to know how many wills contain provisions that are no longer valid or that clearly are no longer the last wish of the deceased. I know a friend who had a terrible marriage, got divorced, remarried, and had a very happy second marriage. He did not review his will, and when he died his first wife was still the sole heir to quite a substantial estate.

I have a very wealthy friend who believes you should always "skip one generation." That means you bequeath your assets to the grandchildren not to your children. Your children in turn bequeath their assets to their grandchildren. You can discuss this with an expert if you want to consider it. I applied this advice only to a smallish portion of my estate.

Do not rule from your grave! I personally believe in this rule and have applied this rule to my own estate planning. What do I mean by this? It simply means that you should not have ridiculous terms in your will that instruct the executor to carry out your wishes even years after your death. It becomes a real struggle to make practical sense out of all these weird conditions.

Examples are the following:

- Your husband or wife inherits your share of the estate, but if he or she remarries within a period of five years after your death, half of the inheritance is to be transferred to a trust for such and such beneficiaries.

- You leave a sum of money to an organization on condition that a specific clause in their constitution will not be amended in the three years following your death.

In general, avoid long-term provisions in your will; it is in many cases not feasible and totally impractical to carry out those wishes. Do not rule from the grave. Hopefully you will be busy with other things.

Do not use your will to punish your children for things you clearly did not succeed to teach them in their upbringing. Be objective and above all be fair. Do not have your memory tarnished by feelings of unfairness by any one of your heirs. Apply the principle of equity.

On the other hand, do not hesitate to use a trust or similar structure when you know there could be a problem if the inheritance is directly in the heir's name. The trust deed in this case is the guideline by which the trust is managed on behalf of the heir.

This will especially apply in the case of mentally handicapped people. This handicap can take many forms, but you should know best when it should apply.

As indicated above, the trust deed will determine how this trust is to be managed on behalf of your heir. So the terms and guidelines of the trust deed should be very clear, simple, practical, and enforceable. I know of cases where there are really impractical provisions in trust deeds, and the trustees find it very difficult to manage the trust properly. Choose trustees you really trust, and then give them absolute discretion to handle the affairs of the trust in the best possible way. Trustees that you have faith in their abilities and that you trust with wide discretionary powers are in my view your best solution. What is an unwise solution is to come up with a trust deed where you think you have covered all the possibilities and eventualities. The future is simply too difficult to forecast. Don't try to do it. Let your trustees manage the trust taking into account the business environment at that particular stage.

Having said that, I still think there should be some basic guidelines for the trustees. One of the provisions should be to have an annual audit on the affairs of the trust. I think it helps to remind even your (trusted) trustees to properly apply their minds to the affairs of the trust. This should naturally result in proper accounting of the transactions of the trust. It could also assist to have the income tax affairs of the trust up to date and in compliance with possible tax amendments. The key is to appoint trustees you fully trust and then allow them to also use their discretion. A combination of basic instructions and absolute discretion by the trustees could, in my opinion, be in the best interest of such an heir.

Estate taxes can be a tricky problem. Not only is the amount payable to be properly and correctly calculated, but the executor also has to find the cash to pay estate taxes. When you do estate planning and you get an expert to help you, always ask the expert to calculate what taxes will be payable.

Keep in mind that legislation in respect of deceased estates change from time to time and could have a major effect on your existing estate planning. Clauses that can be regarded as brilliant under present legislation could prove to be the opposite under changed legislation. This is another reason for at least an annual review of your last will.

I do not believe to be in "muddy schemes" in order to reduce estate taxes. Do not even consider it! This does not mean that you cannot request your adviser to ensure that within the provisions of the applicable legislation, estate taxes are minimized. Sometimes your choice of wording makes a difference. In other instances you can bequeath your assets in a different manner, or use a slightly different structure and still achieve the same goal. Ask your adviser about this, and ensure that you stay within the boundaries of the law but in such a way as to receive the greatest benefits for your deceased estate. Remember, however, that good planning now may turn into bad planning later if the legislation changes.

It sounds so obvious, but ensure (as far as possible) that the expert you use is still in practice and is still up to date with the most recent developments (like decided cases) and legislation. A retired expert is most probably not such a person.

The expert assisting you to do your estate planning should also calculate the probable executor's remuneration and the taxes payable based on this planning. This means that you also have to provide for some cash to pay the taxes, executor's remuneration, and other creditors. So you have to determine what liquid assets will be available on death, or alternatively what assets will be converted into cash. This in turn could have an effect on your decision on what investments to make during you lifetime.

There are financial institutions that will assist in your estate planning and draw up your will, free of charge. In turn the financial institution expects to be appointed as executor of your deceased estate. Far from implying that these people are not experts in their field and are not objective in their advice to you, my personal preference is to pay for this expert and make your own choice of the appointment of the executor.

When it comes to the choice of an executor, use an expert with a lot of practical experience and who seems to have effective administrative abilities. This is important as the dealings with the relevant authorities can sometimes be really taxing. There could be a lot of red tape involved and many forms to be submitted correctly and timely. Your executor must be capable of dealing effectively and swiftly with any problem that arises out of the administration process. The alternative is the administration of an estate that just drags on and on, disrupting the lives of all the people that are affected by this deceased estate.

When an executor for the deceased estate is appointed, it is normally from the following:

- An expert that meets the requirements as set out above

- An expert jointly with a family member (surviving spouse or child, for example)

- A financial institution like a bank

- A financial institution jointly with a family member

- A family member (e.g., spouse or child) with the power of assumption, i.e., the right to appoint an expert

- A combination of the above

A financial institution like a bank would normally have a division within the organization that specializes on the administration of deceased estates.

There is a lot to be said in favor of appointing a family member (usually one of the beneficiaries) jointly with a financial institution or an expert to act as executors. This makes it more personal, acts as a link between the heirs and the executors, and in general makes it easier to communicate the progress with the administration of the deceased estate.

An heir (beneficiary) or more than one heir or beneficiaries can be appointed to act as executors with the power of assumption. This means that the executor can appoint and pay an expert to assist the executor to properly perform the executor's duties.

Let's discuss the executor's fees (executor's remuneration). Executor's fees are the fees that are payable by the estate for carrying out the wishes of the testator and properly administrate the deceased estate under the existing applicable legislation. Legislation prescribes maximum executor's fees but does not preclude anybody to negotiate lower fees. As an example, it is possible to negotiate to pay only 60 percent of the prescribed fees. You could determine in your will that executor's

fees will only be say 60 percent of the then payable executor's fees. However, you must bear in mind that the appointed executor might decide not to accept the executorship under such a condition.

Please also remember that an heir can reject any inheritance if the inheritance is coupled with conditions that are unacceptable to the heir. Nobody can force you to accept an inheritance or accept to act as an executor of a deceased estate. Because of this it is important that the testator provide for an alternative should that happens.

Is it necessary to remind you that the properly signed will should be kept in a safe place in your safe or with a bank?

Do not make the mistake of neglecting to make updates part of your will – either by drawing up a new will or adding a codicil (supplement). Updates jotted down in your Last Will File should be avoided. Whatever you want to say, say it in your will in plain, clear language.

It is an excellent idea to gather all the important documents relating to your will and put it in your Last Will File. Some of the documents could be:

- Original last will

- Title deeds of fixed assets

- Share certificates

- Life and other insurance policies

- Particulars of mortgage bonds

- Guarantees issued

- Details of unlisted companies, including loan accounts

- Contracts and agreements in which you are involved

- Bank and bank accounts particulars

- Investments

- Details of investment managers and their portfolios

- Liabilities and loans

- Copy of latest personal income tax returns

- Copy of latest personal balance sheets

- Firearm licenses

- Registration documents of vehicles

- Particulars of safe deposit boxes and authorization to open these boxes

In summary: Ensure this is what you really want your Last Will to be. Do not have impractical conditions in your Last Will. Do not try to rule from the grave. Write your Last Will in plain clear language and update it regularly. Keep a proper Last Will File—somebody will be very grateful for this.

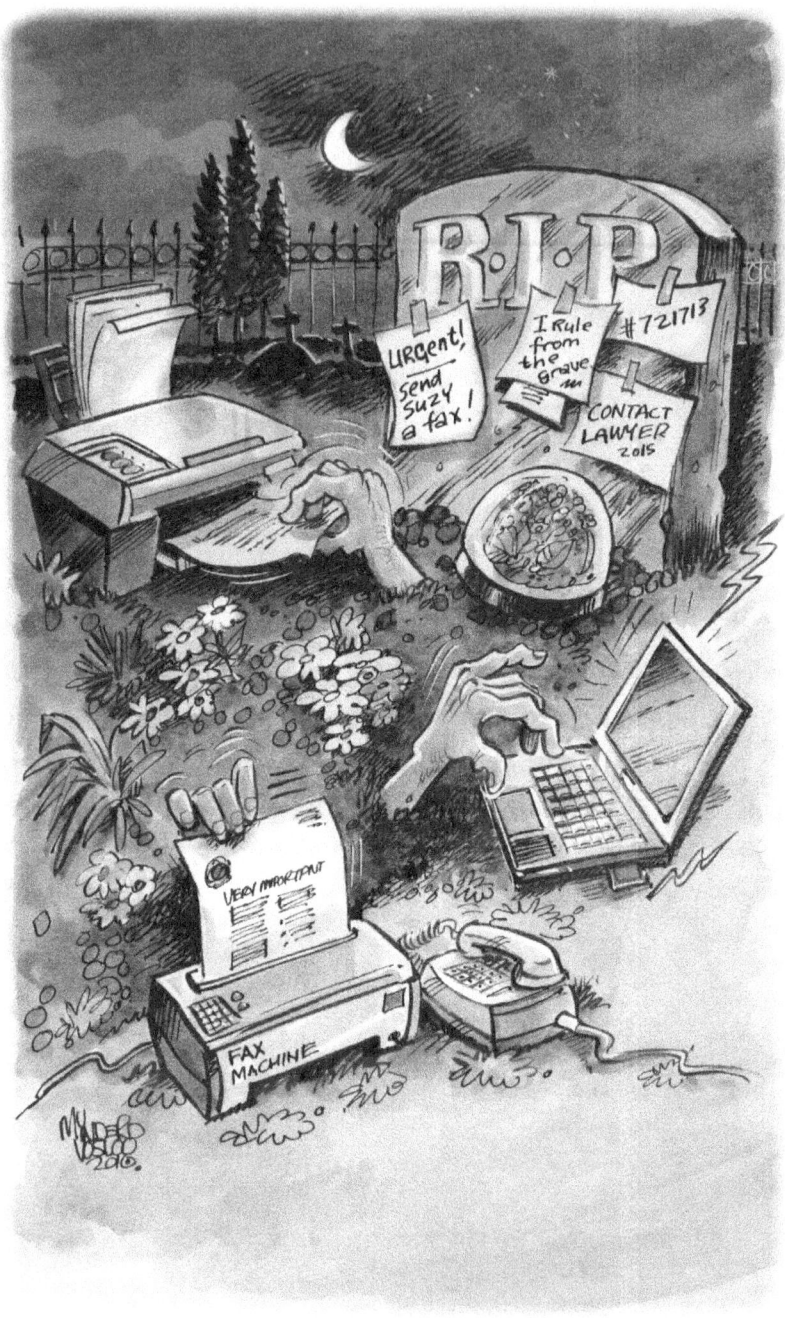

CHAPTER 8

DRIVING YOUR CAR

With us older people it becomes a bone of contention whether we still should be driving our car. When do we become not only a safety hazard to ourselves but to the many other people using the public roads. Do I still see well enough, hear well enough, and are my reflexes still good enough to handle a big car at reasonable high speeds or in bad weather conditions? Even driving at night can be a challenge. I know it is wonderful to still be able to drive your own car. It gives you a sense of freedom and independence.

It is amazing how so many of us older people have the perception that we are really good drivers. More than that, most of us think that we are much better than the average driver. As a matter of fact, most of us would still be racing competitively if it were not for our nagging wives telling us how poorly we drive and that we are too old to race in any case.

Recently I heard about an elderly woman whose driver's license had expired. She went to renew it again, but the officer did a simple eye test and encouraged her to go to an eye specialist for a proper evaluation. The eye specialist was not happy with the outcome of the tests and strongly advised the woman not to drive. Later, it came to light that this woman's eyesight had been seriously impaired for more than a year. So for more than a year she was driving her car and risked getting involved in serious accidents. Sometimes there were a number of her friends in the car. Her excuse was that she was not ready to give up her independence.

When you go for your annual medical checkup, it is worth your while to also have your sight, your hearing, and your reflexes tested. Be proactive. Do not wait until a traffic officer has to tell you that you need to have urgent medical attention.

If you have somebody who will give you an honest opinion on your driving abilities and habits, you can easily act proactively. This person can observe objectively and give an honest opinion on your driving abilities. Whatever the outcome of this is, act on it. Get a second opinion if necessary.

If night driving is a problem, try to avoid driving at night time altogether. If this is not possible, do limit it to the bare minimum.

I use my GPS (global positioning system) a lot. I shall never drive to an unknown destination without my GPS. In this way I know exactly:

- How to get there

- Where to turn

- Expected time of arrival at my destination

- How far I am from my destination

- The availability of parking garages

- Places of interest near your present destination or anywhere else

- The location of hospitals, supermarkets, restaurants, or filling stations, etc.

It is very comforting to being told where to turn off, especially at night, under foggy conditions, or where the visibility in general is poor.

You should never talk on your cell phone (mobile phone) while you are driving. You cannot concentrate on your driving while talking on your cell phone. Show me a motorist that is driving badly and irresponsibly, and I'll show a motorist talking on a cell phone while driving. I do know that there are sophisticated hands-free sets available. Even so, you must be very careful not to lose your concentration even when using these hands-free sets.

If you have to make or receive a call, ask the person to hang on for a moment or two, drive to a place where you can safely turn off the road, stop, and take or make your call. It seems that no one can concentrate on the traffic around you and simultaneously have a violent argument over the phone. Do not talk on your cell phone while driving. Period. In addition to the fact that it is illegal, it is very dangerous.

Make sure you are a member of one of the road assistance services. If you have a breakdown with your car, you can expect to be assisted within minutes rather than hours. In South Africa it is dangerous and unsafe to wait until help arrives, especially in certain areas. Fortunately there are systems on sale that would prevent a tire blow up if you would get a flat tire. The system allows driving for a number of kilometers where you can safely change the tire.

It is necessary that you service your vehicle regularly. The idea is to lower the chances where you would be with a breakdown in an area you do not want to be. If you are going to drive for long distances, get somebody to help you. Stop regularly, stretch your legs, and try not to get overly tired. When you stop, stop in a secure or safe place like they have at most fuel stations.

Driving under the influence of alcohol is completely out. The story is told about a man that was reeling drunk who was getting into his car when a policeman came up and asked, "You're not going to drive that car, are you?" The man replied, "Certainly I am going to drive." Anybody can see I am in no condition to walk."[4]

There is no reason to drive if you have used alcohol. Do not even consider it. I know many people who would not even consider taking any alcohol at all if they know they have to drive. It does not matter whether you believe that the alcohol content in your blood is less than the legally allowable limit. This is not the point. The point is you should not drive if you have used any alcohol. Alcohol reduces your driving ability. Don't drink and drive. It is just not worth it.

Unfortunately certain medications can have the same effect on us as alcohol. The same rule applies. If the medication makes you drowsy, if it affects your reflexes, do not drive. With all proper medication comes a leaflet, giving you the results of years of development and research. It will clearly spell out the possible effects of taking that medicine. It is normally the following: "The use of this medicine leads to drowsiness which is aggravated by the simultaneous intake of alcohol". Please take this warning very seriously.

If there is the slightest indication that the medication would affect your driving ability, do not drive. Ask someone else to drive, get a taxi, sleepover, or whatever. Just do not drive.

---

4 Winston K Pendleton, *2121 Funny Stories and How to Tell Them* (Missouri: The Bethany Press, 1977), 51.

A group of senior citizens are discussing their various ailments in a nursing home one afternoon.

"I am so feeble that I can hardly lift this cup of coffee," said one old lady.

"Tell me about it. My cataracts are so bad I can't even see what is on my plate," replied another.

"I can't turn my head because of the arthritis in my neck."

"My joints are so stiff and swollen that I have difficulty going to the bathroom at night."

"My blood pressure pills make me dizzy," another old lady said.

"I guess that's the price you pay for getting old," sighed an old man slowly shaking his head.

"Well it's not that bad," said one woman cheerfully. "At least we can still drive."[5]

Ultimately, each of us will come to the point where it will be irresponsible of us to drive our own car. Not only could we become a danger to ourselves but also to the other people on the road.

I can imagine that this could have a big impact on your life because you were accustomed to come and go as you please. You could also feel that your independence is also heavily impeded. It is here when we need to make a mind shift. Not being able to drive your car anymore can only have a big impact on your life if you allow it to do so. Do not allow this to

5 Shelly Klein, *The Little Book of Senior Moments* (London: Michael O'Hara Books, 2008), 45.

get you into the darkest valleys of depression but see it positively as a new phase in your life. No matter how difficult it might be to believe this, it's not the end of the world if you cannot drive your car anymore. There are a number of alternatives to consider that could make life much easier for you:

- Appoint a chauffeur if you can afford it.

- If you cannot afford a chauffeur, get a few of your best friends together and pay for the chauffeur jointly.

- Ask one of your younger friends to drive your car.

- Get a student to drive you to concerts, etc. Most probably you can remunerate the student in part or in full by buying a ticket for the student and perhaps a meal at the venue.

- Most car rental companies offer a service to transport you from point to point. Some even specialize to take you to specific events, and after the event, collect you and take you home. If more than one person shares the cost, it could be more affordable.

There are also many advantages if you do not drive your car yourself:

- You can really relax and need not worry about getting everyone home again.

- As you will not be driving, you may take alcohol if that is your inclination.

- You need not worry about driving at night or in foreign places.

- You need not worry about parking as you would normally be dropped or picked up right in front of the building where the event is taking place.

Please talk to your insurer if you are going to use the car in these ways and ensure that your insurance would cater for any eventuality in this regard and that the insurance coverage is adequate. Also ask for third-party insurance. I hope you would never have to make use of this insurance, but if you need the insurance, you must be adequately covered.

It is not the end of the world if you cannot drive your car anymore. Make the mind shift and enjoy this phase of your life. Not being able to drive your car anymore is no excuse not to live a quality life.

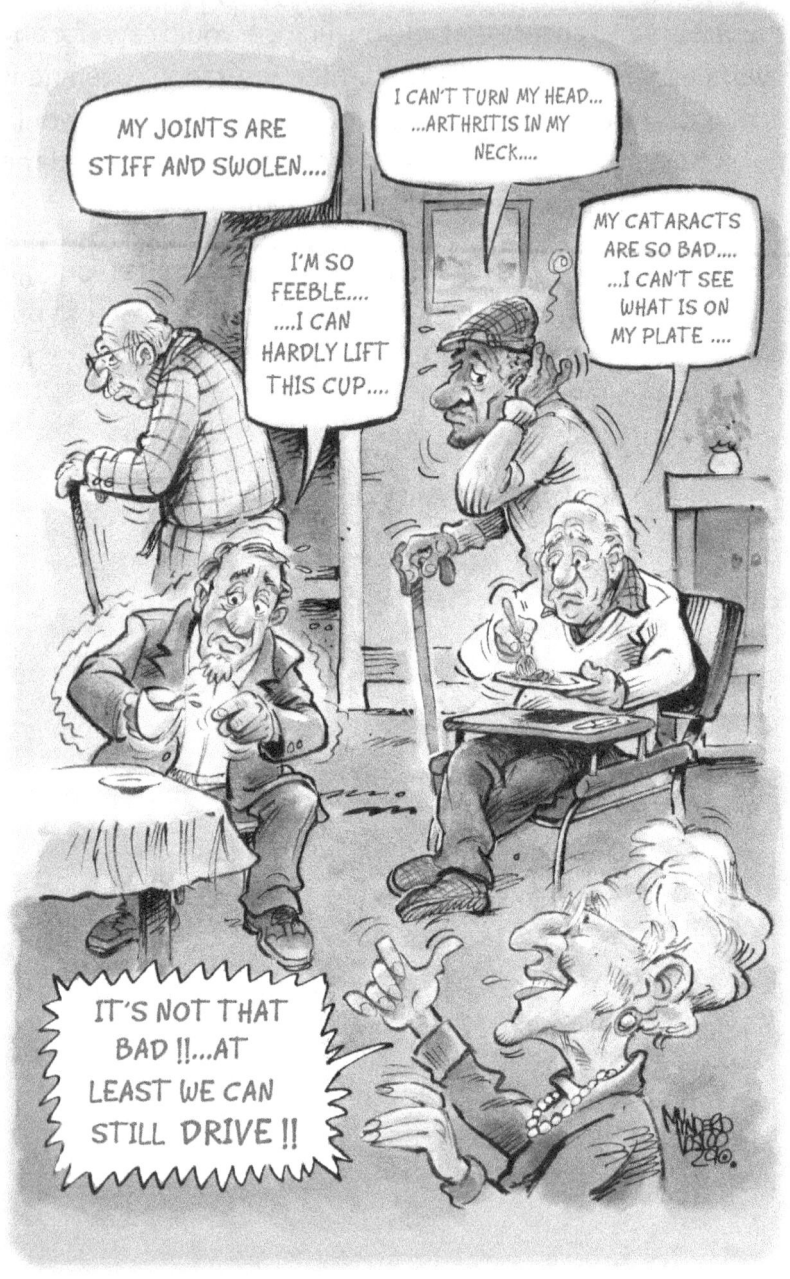

CHAPTER 9

CONTRACTS AND AGREEMENTS

"It is because of ethics that civilized man developed the attitude that it is fairer to rob a man with a contract than with a gun."[6]

From time to time all of us will be confronted to sign some or other agreement or contract. When this happens it is nice to have some basic guidelines to ensure that we do not do something stupid or irresponsible. It is therefore necessary for us to discuss certain basic guidelines when it comes to contracts or agreements.

The first and cardinal guideline: Do not sign any contract or agreement until you are satisfied that it is in your best interest to sign that contract or agreement. If you are in any doubt whether all the conditions are acceptable to you, do not put your signature on such a document but go for legal advice. It is always best to get legal advice before you sign a contract. At that stage you can still request amendments to the contract should that be necessary. At that stage all parties to the agreement are (normally) still friends and would like the transaction to go through.

---

6 Winston K Pendleton, *2121 Funny Stories and How to Tell Them* (Missouri: The Bethany Press, 1977), 175.

Once you have signed a contract it is very difficult to get any amendments to that contract. Moreover, if you then have to involve legal people, it can be very expensive. It can also become very time consuming and stressful. The best time to obtain legal advice is before you put your signature to anything. Even if the legal costs seem a little scary, it will never the less be much cheaper than trying to amend or nullify a contract afterwards.

Talking about the legal fees. This man made a deal with his lawyer. "I'll give you a hundred dollars a month to do my worrying for me," he said "That's a deal," said the lawyer. "Where's the hundred?" His client replied, "That's your first worry."[7]

If the conditions and terms of the contract do not bring about a win-win situation for all the parties to the contract, it is a contract that normally won't last. Such a contract cannot be conducive to a long-term business relationship and will probably be terminated as soon as legally possible.

Please note that nobody on this planet can legally force you to sign any document. Of course I am not talking where somebody could force you to sign a document at gunpoint. In South Africa, you can only be compelled to sign a document by an order of the High Court.

Apart from an order of the High Court, you need not sign any document you do not wish to. Never sign a document until you have read it through thoroughly and until you really understand each clause of the contract. Do not hesitate to get any legal advice you need before you sign the contract. Even if you are a lawyer, if you're unsure about something, ask a

---

7 Winston K Pendleton, *2121 Funny Stories and How to Tell Them* (Missouri: The Bethany Press, 1977), 119.

colleague. The cost for proper advice may seem high, but it is much cheaper than a costly lawsuit later.

If you are pressed to sign the contract as soon as possible for whatever reason, always resist that pressure and take your time to properly read and understand the document. Except maybe when you have to give permission for an emergency operation, it is unlikely that any contract is so important that you have to sign that document immediately. If you are worried about any ambiguity in the document, get it corrected in plain clear language. If you are told that the contract stipulates one thing, but in reality the other party means something different, do not sign! Beware, problems are looming. Insist that the document be amended so that it says exactly what is meant and what is the intention of all parties. It is unacceptable that legal words or phrases are used in a contract that you do not understand. Insist that these wording be changed to clear plain language. A good contract is a contract that is drawn up in such a way and in plain and clear language as to clearly spell out exactly what the intentions of the parties to the contract really are.

Sometimes you do not act on behalf of yourself or in your personal capacity, but, for example, on behalf of a trust or a company. In this case, you should always have signed minutes of the resolution of the trustees (in the case of a trust) or a resolution of the directors of the company (in the case of a company), in which you are authorized to act on behalf of the trust or the company and are authorized to sign that specific document. This should prevent a possible dispute later whether you really had the authority to have signed that contract. Normally certified minutes authorizing you to sign the specific documents are attached to the contract.

Get a reputation that you do not sign a contract without investigating all the facts properly. If you have a reputation that you sign everything that is put before you, it is no compliment.

It is obvious that you should at least have a proper legible copy of the final contract with all the related documents and minutes where applicable. These will be placed in a safe place.

I normally make a one-page summary of any contract I am a party to. On this one page (and if I say one page, I really mean one page) summary all the salient features of the contract are highlighted. A contract for the rent of property, for example, can be summarized as follows:

- Brief description of property

- Name of tenant and landlord

- Commencement date of contract

- End date. Option to renew? If YES, at what rate and explain the conditions?

- Amount of rent per period

- Escalation, and escalation date and percentage of escalation

- Perhaps a note on the building's insurance

Most cell phones (mobile phones) have the facility to enable you to copy this one pager into a file on the phone. The same can be done with summarized budgets, income statements, and balance sheets. If you have to kill some time at the airport or at the doctor's consulting rooms, you can productively use your time by reading through these summaries. Your friends will be very surprised on how well you know your business.

Follow the simple guidelines I have given above, it is practical and it works. If you follow the guidelines above before you sign a contract, it is highly unlikely that you will end up with a contract that is really a headache and has the potential of large future legal costs.

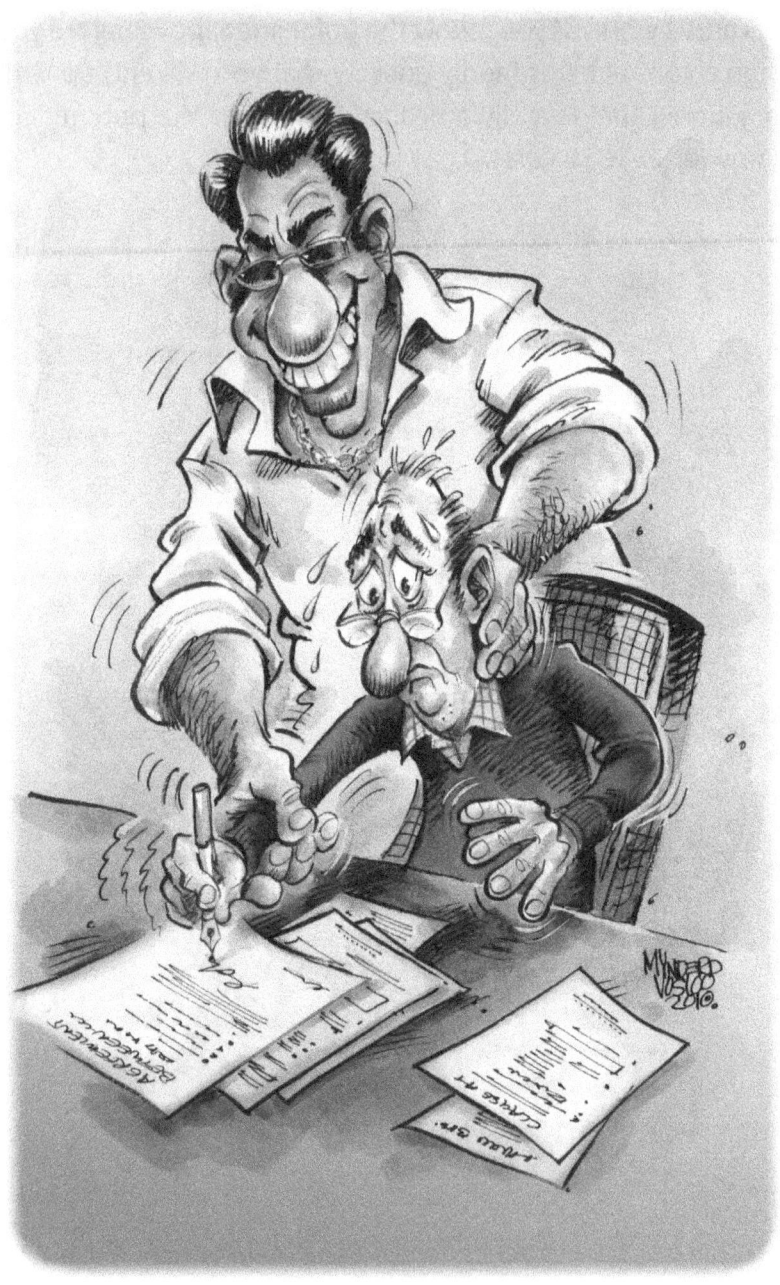

CHAPTER 10

EXERCISES AND SOCIAL LIFE

Remember, even a brisk walk in a safe environment is much better than just sitting in front of the television set. If you're older and not as healthy, it is very important to exercise under the guidance and control of you medical practitioner. This can also be done under the watchful eye of a person who specialized in biokinetics.

On a lighter note actress and comedian Ellen De Generes wrote, "You must keep it in shape. My grandmother started to walk five miles a day when she was sixty. She's ninety-seven today, and we don't know where she is."[8]

When spring is in the air, don't get out and start to exercise like a fanatic. This can do more harm than good. Ask your medical practitioner or your personal trainer to work out the appropriate exercises and go about these exercises with enthusiasm. Exercise on a regular basis. Try not to skip any session. Once you have skipped a session it is easier to skip another session, and before you know, you are back in front of the tele-

---

8 Shelly Klein, *The Little Book of Senior Moments* (London: Michael O'Hara Books, 2008), 52

vision set. You must persevere and keep exercising. You will never regret it. It also gives you a sense of accomplishment.

If you still participate in tennis, bowls, golf, or any sport whatsoever, carry on doing it. It is wonderful therapeutic activity and very good for your health (especially if done with insight and moderation). It also can be an important part of your social life. I know a group of friends that get together every week after bowling for a barbeque. Needless to say no one wants to miss out on this nice social activity; the attendance is almost always 100 percent.

It is quite funny that most of us older people think that their hearing is also 100 percent. You know as well as I do what a struggle it can be to follow conversations in a crowded noisy room or in a restaurant where the sounds come from all directions. I am told that the younger you start using a hearing aid, the easier it is to adapt to it. I am going to a good audiologist next week. Should not you do the same?

A seventy-five year old man goes the doctor for a physical and a few days later the doctor sees him walking down the street with a stunning young lady on his arm and a huge smile on his face. A couple more days passed and the old man returns to the doctor's surgery. After he has again examined the elderly man, the doctor writes him a prescription and said, "You're really doing well, aren't you?" The patient replied, "Just doing what you said, doctor: "Get a hot mamma and be cheerful. That's what you have told me and that is what I have done." The doctor said, "Actually I said you have a heart murmur and need to be careful. Now while you are here, why don't we check your hearing?"[9]

---

9 Shelly Klein, *The Little Book of Senior Moments* (London: Michael O'Hara Books, 2008), 31.

Should there be no social activities where you live, take the initiative and start something. The social life will not fall from the sky. The world does not owe you a life of nice social activities. What about water aerobics that can be part of your exercise program? What about a dance club, a bridge club, or become friends of the steam engine. Don't forget cultural activities like music evenings, meetings on the newest trends in literature, or Bible study groups. What about a get together for bird watchers? It is not important what you do. What is important is that you do something.

If there are social activities, participate in it. Do not just be a "sleeping member" (literally and figuratively). The key is to participate.

If special events are coming to your town or city, like exhibits, performing artists, choirs, operas, or whatever, organize some friends and go together. This is good fun and contributes to a quality lifestyle.

Get a few friends together and go to the cinema. Just do something. Why don't you go on a golf or bowling tour? It is great fun. If you are fond of fly fishing, why do you not you go for a trout weekend. Better still, don't go over the weekend because it is more expensive. Take a midweek break that is less expensive. Just do something. Get out of your comfort zone. Get away from your television set.

Use your GPS (global positioning system) to drive to these places. With the GPS it is easy to find these places. I also have a GPS on my cell phone. Because of the small dial it is not as easy to use when driving but ideal when you are walking in a foreign city. Just a piece of advice: Before you download the GPS maps on your cell phone, first determine the cost per month of this facility.

For many people the cherry on top is to travel abroad. There are three important guidelines you must take note off:

- The first guideline is: TRAVEL LIGHT!

- The second guide line is: travel light.

- The third guideline is: travel light.

I know you can read, and I know you understand what I am saying, but somehow deep down the traveler abroad ignore this guideline. If you can really travel light, it can make such a difference in getting around easily and enjoying your trip.

When we pack for overseas, many of us argue more or less as follows: Well, it is summertime, let me take summer clothing. But what if it gets colder? So let me pack some warm clothing. The new jacket I bought will be ideal, so let me take it. That classy dress I bought the other day will suit me just fine. Ultimately we are struggling to keep below the allowed weight allowance for our baggage. Fortunately, there are limitations on weight and size of luggage or I would not know how large and heavy our suitcases would have been.

If you travel to different countries abroad, you have to collect all your bags and go through customs at point of entry. In most cases, you have to handle your bags yourself. It is unbelievable that you find many people with such big and heavy suitcases that it really takes a strong person to handle them. The irony is that those people cannot handle their own baggage easily. All you achieve by having these heavy and bulky suitcases is to injure some handler's back (or yours).

The answer is obvious: travel light.

If you go on any tour make sure what the physical demands for that tour would be. I know an elderly lady who went on a safari in Africa not knowing that the intention was to rough it a bit and required a reasonable level of fitness. What should have been a dream holiday became a nightmare.

Keep your hand luggage within the requirements of the airlines. Ensure that it is easily manageable. I prefer the type with small wheels that you can pull around easily. This makes it easy to handle especially in the long corridors at the airports and the long queues at passport controls. Alternatively, I use a small day backpack that I carry on my back. I've found it easy to handle. This is no good for anybody with back problems.

In my hand luggage I usually also keep the following:

- My travel documents.

- My toothbrush and razor:

- My chronic medication (with a copy of the doctor's prescription). I take the doctor's prescription with in case I will need extra medication or in case medics have to determine what medication I take. Especially in the Far East your medication can be mistaken for drugs.

- My extra pair of reading glasses.

- One set of clean underwear and socks.

- Travel insurance documents.

- A copy of my passport (another copy is in my other luggage). If you lose your passport and have to apply at a foreign office mission, it is a little easier if you have a copy of your passport and other identification.

I keep my chronic medicine with me, so that even if my baggage gets lost, I can still take my chronic medication regularly.

There are also suitcases available that are self-driven similar to some golf carts. I have not yet tried one of these.

Be sure you leave a copy of your itinerary with someone at home, as well as a copy of your medical insurance. If the people at home need to trace you, it is quite easy if they have a proper itinerary. If you have to be hospitalized and for some reason lost the medical insurance, you could phone home and get the particulars.

Do not even consider leaving home without proper travel and medical insurance. It is not even negotiable! Make sure your medical insurance is adequate. The medical costs abroad can be really high. I once had to undergo two emergency operations in a foreign country. The cost thereof was astronomical. Fortunately, I had proper and adequate medical insurance. If you use certain credit cards to pay your travel expenses, you will automatically receive certain travel and medical insurance free of charge. Be very sure that the insurance is adequate and cover all types of emergencies.

For many, traveling abroad is an exciting experience. Follow the above guidelines and make it also a memorable one.

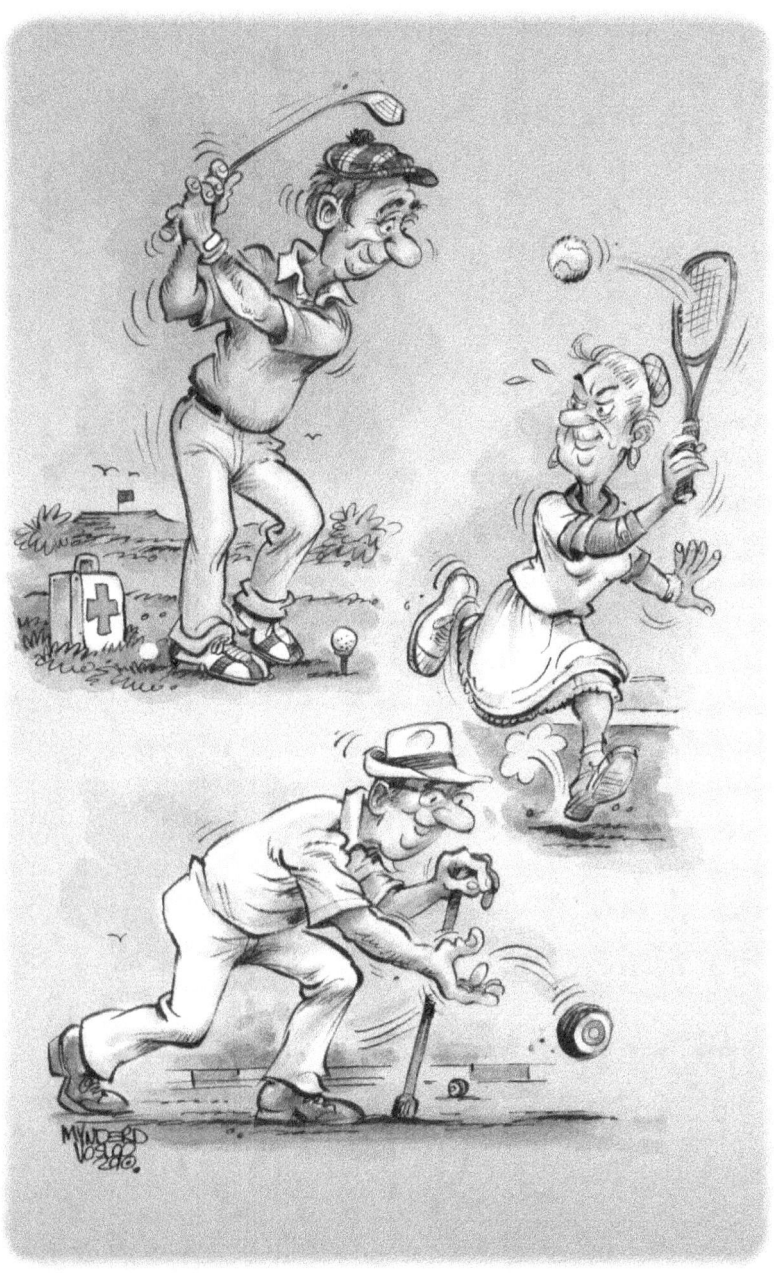

CHAPTER 11

YOU MUST (STILL) HAVE A PURPOSE IN LIFE

If you would ask some of your older friends whether they still have a specific purpose in life, you might be shocked at the answer. There are so many people out there who do not have a dream they would like to fulfill. Some would even tell you they are too old to chase a dream. What nonsense. I have read many books on this subject and never ever did I come across anything that indicates an age restriction on when to stop dreaming.

One should always have a purpose in life or more than one purpose. You must still have a dream you would like to chase regardless of your age. To have a purpose in life makes life that extra bit of interesting. To chase that dream is always worth the effort. Because it is not in the fulfillment of the dream that life is worth living, but the journey to attain that purpose is really what life is all about.

You should never stop having a purpose in life. You should never stop having a dream and chasing after it. Nobody is ever too old to have a dream. It does not matter what your dream is, as long as you still have one despite your age. It also does not matter whether your dream is little or big. What is big for one person might be little for another.

Johann Wolfgang von Goethe advised "Dream no small dreams for they have no power to move the hearts of men."

Of course you must be very practical about your dream. If you want to climb Mt. Kilamanjaro, you must still be physically strong enough to do just that. On the other hand do not use this as an excuse to set yourself little dreams. The idea is for you to reach that goal you'll have to put in that little extra, to go that extra mile, and to really be challenged. Only you will know if your goal was set high enough. Your dream should be achievable but with some extra effort.

But most important of all, you must have a dream!

Once you have determined what you dream is, write down the steps you need to take to get you there. Tick off each step as you progress until you finally have reached your goal. Enjoy this satisfaction of achieving what you set out to do, bask a little in this sense of fulfillment, and then map your new goal, your new dream.

Why is it absolutely necessary to have a dream to pursue? It makes life tick. Apart from other values that make life worthwhile, it gives you a new purpose in life. It keeps you focusing and striving. It gives you a sense of being worth it.

What do other people say about goal setting? I read the following that I would like to share with you: "Goal-setting techniques are used by top-level athletes, successful business people, and achievers in all fields."[10] Goal-setting was therefore an important ingredient of the success recipe of many achievers.

Do not even try to tell me that this does not apply to older people because it cannot be further from the truth. This is a

_____

10 Editorial article, *"Golden Rules of Goal Setting,"* Mind Tools, http:/www.mindtools.com (August 2009).

universal law and is applicable to all of us. This law cannot distinguish between young and old, what the color of your skin is, or how successful or unsuccessful you have been in the past.

The attainment of modest targets will convince you that this technique works like a charm! Try it, and I'm sure you'll be surprised how well it works.

Another important issue in this regard is that your goal setting should meet the following requirements. Your goal should be:

- Very specific

- Achievable

- Measurable

- Expressed in positive language.

It is of utmost importance that your goal should be very specific. Let us say your goal is to make a lot of money in the next number of years. Your goal should not be: "I want to make a lot of money in the next number of years."

Your goal should be, "I will make $3 million (or whatever amount) before December 31, 2013."

Your goal should be achievable, but it must take you out of your comfort zone. It must stretch your resources. It must force you to walk the extra mile. It must make you fire on all cylinders.

Your goal should be measurable. The goal "I will make $3 million before December 31, 2013," is absolutely measurable. You know exactly how much you want to accumulate and by when. A very good way to get to your goal is to break the goal into small measurable steps that eventually leads to the major goal. Decide what should be achieved with each step. Measure yourself at each step and determine if you still are on course.

Your goal should be expressed in positive language. You should never state your goal as: I hope I can have about $3 million in the next five years. No, your goal should be stated positively: I will make $3 million before December 31, 2013.

Your goal will not necessarily be about money. There are so many other things that your goal can be:

- Write that book

- Go on a trip around the world

- Go on an extended safari

- Go on a hiking trip in Italy

- Learn to speak a foreign language

- Take lessons in sculpturing

- Lower your golf handicap

- Become the bowling champion of your club

If your goal is to become the president of a cultural society, and you succeed in achieving that, please do not fall in the trap of making long and uninteresting speeches that no one really wants to hear. This story is about a speaker that was longwinded and dry. As he went on and on, people gradually slipped out until at last the audience had dwindled down to a single man in the front row. "I wish to pause here, my friend," the speaker said to this man, "to thank you for your courtesy in remaining to hear all of my speech." "Oh, that's all right," said the man. " I don't need any thanks. I am the next speaker."[11]

Seriously, whatever your goal is you should never stop to dream. Strive for higher and better.

I quote again from the article above: "By setting sharp, clearly defined goals, you can measure and take pride in the achievement of those goals. You can see forward progress in what might previously have seemed a long pointless grind. By setting goals, you will raise your self-confidence as you recognize your ability and competence in achieving these goals that you have set."[12]

Get yourself a reason why you want to jump out of bed every morning! When you have achieved your goal it is time to set your next and more challenging goal.

---

11 Winston K Pendleton, *2121 Funny Stories and How to Tell Them* (Missouri: The Bethany Press, 1977), 403.
12 Editorial article, *"Golden Rules of Goal Setting,"* Mind Tools, http:/www.mindtools.com (August 2009).

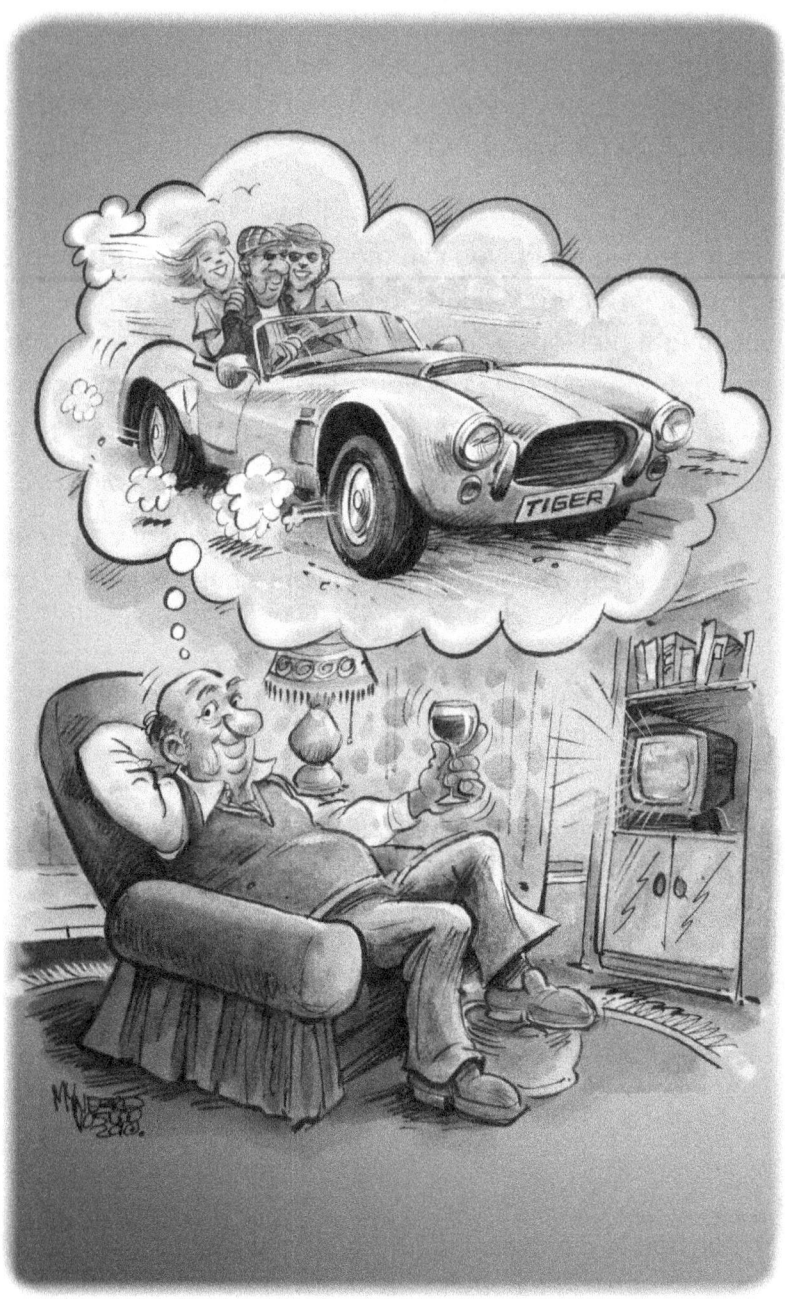

CHAPTER 12

PERSONAL HYGIENE

The word *hygiene* is derived from the name of the Greek goddess Hygeia, the goddess of health. The concept of hygiene is a centuries-old concept. To frequent a public bath was a part of the ancient Roman culture. Larger and smaller public baths were quite common in the later Roman period. Both the Hindu and Muslim cultures placed strong emphasis on personal hygiene since the earliest times.

Personal hygiene is very different from person to person. It depends much on the culture you grew up in, the family you are part of and what your own perception is what your personal hygiene should be. Personal hygiene includes not only the cleanliness of your body, but also includes proper skincare, regular visits to the dentist, and your overall health through proper diet and a healthy lifestyle. Good personal hygiene can help you to lead a quality lifestyle and allow you to be acceptable to the society at large. There is surely nothing more obnoxious than a person afflicted with bad breath. One involuntarily associates it with badly discolored teeth and unhealthy gums. Bad body smells are simply not acceptable.

It would appear to me that older people should be very mindful as far as their personal hygiene is concerned. As a matter of fact it is really at this stage of your life that you want this aspect of your life to be in order. We often get the opposite—older people are no longer so meticulous about personal hygiene, their appearance, and their general appearance is often neglected. It is so unfortunate that this should happen because it is so easy to improve this aspect of our lives, especially because there are a lot of effective solutions on the market.

Since childhood I have the perception that older people sometimes have peculiar body smells. Whether it is so or not, you can easily handle this with all the nice body deodorants and sprays that are available on the market. The important thing is to be aware of this, and to know that you can easily take care of it.

It is unfortunately also true that a man's hair at a certain age grows better out of your nostrils and your ears than on your head. This is just a fact. Nobody, however, appreciates a lush growth of hair out of your nostrils or ears. Remove that hair—nobody wants to see it. Do it regularly every week at a fixed time; it works best that way.

Men, you have every reason to shave regularly and properly every day. On a lighter note, the whiskey-smelling barber was shaving the minister and not doing a very good job. Suddenly the razor slipped and the minister was bleeding from a bad cut. "Now you see," said the minister, "what comes from drinking too much.""Yes, sir," said the barber sympathetically, "drinking sure does make the skin tender, don't it?"[13]

---

13 Winston K Pendleton, *2121 Funny Stories and How to Tell Them* (Missouri: The Bethany Press, 1977), 55.

Good care of your fingernails is obvious. Women often spend a lot of time and money to manicure their nails. It is important that your hands are well cared for as you use it quite a lot, and some of us even when communicating and when talking over the phone. Some people's toenails are really very unattractive and badly manicured. If yours fall into this category, do something about it.

All the above are important elements of a well-groomed appearance. There is no reason why at any stage of your life your personal hygiene and appearance must be neglected. If you know your personal hygiene is good, and you are well groomed, it gives you much more confidence in your contact with other people.

Sometimes there might be an excuse for not being well groomed. The man said to the bum on the street who had asked him for a handout, "You would stand more of a chance of getting a job if you would shave and clean yourself up." The bum replied, "Yes sir. I found that out years ago."[14]

Unfortunately it would appear that many older people are unable to see the dirty spots on their clothes. Ensure that your clothes are fresh and clean. You should always look at your very best whether you are going to a big occasion or just a small get together. Avoid being overdressed. Dress for the occasion. You dress differently for church than for golf or a music concert. If you are well groomed and neatly dressed, you will feel even more welcome and at home. This may lead to further invitations and appointments and special occasions—if you really want it of course.

---

14 Winston K Pendleton, *2121 Funny Stories and How to Tell Them* (Missouri: The Bethany Press, 1977), 39.

Unpleasant or bad breath is something that plagues young and old. Most people are not willing to tell you in your face that you have bad breath; they will avoid you instead. There are really good mouthwashes and even breath rinses on the market that will enable you to get this problem under control. Their manufacturers claim that these washes and rinses effectively remove bacteria, food debris, and dead cells that cause bad breath. Once it is under control, keep it under control. Keep your regular appointment with your dentist. The dentist will not only be looking after your teeth but also after your gums. Infected gums could be part of the problem. Healthy gums are important for your overall health. Discuss this with your dentist.

We should all visit a dermatologist from time to time. In South Africa, with the harsh African sun, it is important to do that regularly. The specialist will examine the skin cancers and stains on the skin and professionally treat or remove what is necessary. Even the general appearance of your skin can be attended to. If you want that done, go for expert advice and help.

General good health is invaluable. If you could supplement good health with a well-groomed appearance and acceptable personal hygiene, you are a well on your way to enjoy a quality lifestyle.

Regular visits to a physician are simply a must. This could lead to extensive blood and other tests. Do not grumble and moan about the inconvenience of some of the tests. Do it! It's really worth it.

This reminds me of the story of the man who just examined by the physician. The doctor said to the patient's wife, "I don't like the looks of your husband." The wife replied, "I don't either, doctor, but he is very kind to the children." [15]

In life there are many issues that can put strain on our relationship with other people. Personal hygiene needs not be one of them!

_____

15 Winston K Pendleton, *2121 Funny Stories and How to Tell Them* (Missouri: The Bethany Press, 1977), 39.

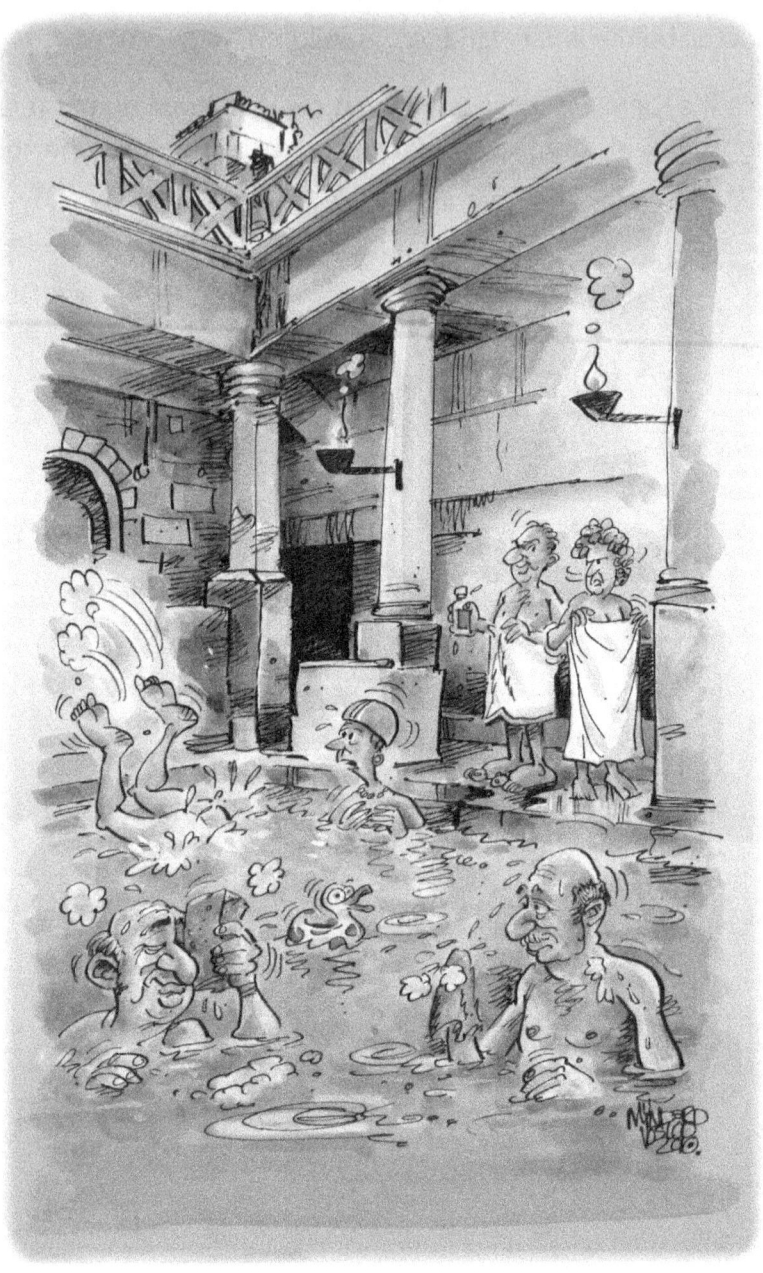

CHAPTER 13

IN CONCLUSION...... YOUR CHECKLIST

This chapter is a summary of what is discussed in this book. It is an easy reference guide to what you will find in each chapter.

Chapter 1 LIVE BEFORE YOU DIE

We must also live until we die. That may sound very obvious to you. Surely we shall all live until we die. However, the question is do we really live until we die or are we merely existing? Going on day after day without a purpose in life. The excuse we use is that we are too old to do exciting things. We are too old to live a meaningful life.

What utter nonsense! So don't sit in front of your television sets and wait for death to come. Get off your butt and run until death overtakes you.

None other than Helen Keller said: "Life is either a daring adventure or nothing." The purpose of this book is to show elderly people that life can still be a daring adventure regardless of your age. Indeed, age is no excuse.

Chapter 2 AGE IS NO EXCUSE

When one looks at the achievements of older people all over the world, one thing is very clear: You are never too old to do what you really want to do. You are never too old to pursue your realistic dream! The people we discuss in this chapter truly lived and will live until they die. They did not and are not using their (old) age as an excuse not to follow their dream. They live life as an exciting adventure.

Grandma Moses, the famous American painter, had her first solo exhibition in New York when she was eighty years old.

Wally Hayward completed the Comrades Marathon in South Africa over a distance of ninety kilometers in nine hours and forty-four minutes at the age of seventy-nine. This was fifty-eight years after he first won this grueling marathon.

Bettie Cilliers Barnard was still a prolific South African painter at the age of ninety-three.

Gadamer, the German philosopher, was still publishing books and article on subjects in his field of excellence when he was ninety-six years old.

Age is no excuse. "Age is an attitude. I am glad I changed mine—should not you?"[16]

Chapter 3 YOU CAN DO SOMETHING ABOUT YOUR MEMORY

When I did a search on the Internet on how to improve your memory I got around 124 million responses! It is clear that there are thousands of ways and many thousands of experts who are of the opinion that you can improve your memory.

---

16 Doris Drummer, Holidays RCI Group, *Autumn* (2010): 33.

I agree wholeheartedly with these people—you and I can improve our memory. We could but need not take difficult and expensive courses to achieve this.

By simply following the guidelines given in this chapter, everyone will be amazed on how much better your memory will be. This will also help you to get things done. The good news is you can do something about your memory. It's easy, it's fun, it costs you nothing extra, and most important of all— it works!

A poor memory can have a very negative effect on your life. Do not spend hours and hours of your valuable life to look for your stuff. Do not accept this situation as a given. You can do something about your memory. Do it!

Chapter 4 EXERCISE THAT BRAIN

To keep our bodies in a healthy condition, we have to exercise regularly and correctly. The saying use it or lose it is very appropriate and very true. The very same principle applies to our brain. We must exercise that brain! It must be done regularly. It must be done on a daily basis. To exercise your brain is as important as exercising you body. Every day (yes, I mean *every* day) your brain must be exposed to something that is complex, difficult to understand, and hopefully sometimes forces your brain to really stretch itself to get a grip on the issue. For me it works well if I tackle something that is totally removed from my own (so-called) field of expertise. Do what works best for you. It is different for everyone. Here is an opportunity to fill your hours with something extraordinary and exciting. Come out of your comfort zone and start doing these brain exercises!

Chapter 5 AND NOW THOSE PILLS

Many senior people are on medication of some sort. Perhaps a bigger number of us are on chronic medication. Can any of you honestly say that you are taking your pills strictly according to the medical practitioner's prescription? A serious problem amongst senior people is that they do not take important prescribed medicine regularly. In many other instances older people are taking excessive medication because they simply cannot remember whether they have already taken their medicine and then just for safety's sake they take the medication again. In this way you can easily take too few pills (underdosage) or too many pills (overdosage). Both overdosage and underdosage can be dangerous for your health and should be avoided at all times.

There are very good reasons why medication should be taken as prescribed. Huge amounts of money are spent on research and development of medicine. Medical practitioners and pharmacists study many years to enable them to prescribe the right quantities that we should take for the benefit of our health. The least we can do is to ensure that we take the medication as prescribed.

The good news is you can easily avoid overdosage or underdosage. There is a whole range of practical and inexpensive methods explained in this chapter you can use to get this right.

Chapter 6 MONEY MATTERS

It seems that older people have become the target of all of the villains, tricksters, and psychopaths of this world. There are too many sad stories where older people have literally lost everything, and now live in the deepest poverty. In this chapter we discuss how can you identify these impostors.

We also discuss inflation and the huge impact inflation has on our investments. Also remember that good advice for a friend might not be good advice for you. Each person's circumstances are unique. Get an expert to help you find the best solutions for your particular financial circumstances.

Never get involved in funny and suspicious schemes to avoid tax—it does not work. In the long run it could result in additional taxes, penalties, and interest payments.

Common sense should prevail:

- If the financial returns are too good to be true, they are too good to be true. Do not touch such an "investment."

- Risk and yield go hand in hand: The higher the yield, the higher the risk. Be careful.

- Follow a conservative investment approach. Rather err on the conservative side.

- The time for taking risks is gone. You should have done that at a much younger age.

Chapter 7 Your last Will

Ensure this is what you really want your Last Will to be. Do not have impractical conditions in your Last Will. Do not try to rule from the grave. Appoint executors you can trust and give them the right to apply their discretion.

Write your Last Will in plain clear language and update it regularly.

In this chapter it is also discussed what to keep on a proper Last Will File. Do it—somebody will be very grateful for this.

Chapter 8 Driving your car

It is amazing how so many of us older people have the perception that we are really good drivers. More than that, most of us think that we are much better than the average driver. As a matter of fact most of us would still be racing if it was not for our nagging wives telling us how poorly we drive and that we are too old to race in any case.

When you go for your annual medical checkup, it is worth your while to also have your sight, your hearing, and your reflexes tested. Be proactive. Do not wait until a traffic officer has to tell you that you need urgent medical attention.

It is not the end of the world if you cannot drive your car anymore. In this chapter we discuss how to make the mind shift and enjoy this phase of your life as well. Not being able to drive your car is no excuse not to live a quality life.

Chapter 9 Contracts and greements

From time to time all of us will be confronted to sign some or other agreement or contract. When this happens it is nice to have some basic guidelines to ensure that we do not do something stupid or irresponsible.

Do not sign any contract or agreement until you are satisfied that it is in your best interest to sign that contract or agreement. If you are in any doubt whether all the conditions are acceptable to you, do not put your signature on such a document and get legal advice. It is always best to get legal advice before you sign a contract. At that stage you can still request amendments to the contract if that is necessary. At that stage all parties to the agreement are (normally) still friends and would like the transaction to go through. Before the contract is signed is the best time to bring in new conditions and have conditions amended.

Once you have signed a contract it is very difficult to get any amendments to that contract. Moreover, if you have to involve legal people, it can be very expensive. It can also become very time consuming and stressful. The best time to obtain legal advice is before you put your signature to anything. Even if the legal costs seem a little scary, it will nevertheless be much cheaper than trying to amend or nullify a contract afterwards.

Chapter 10 EXERCISE AND SOCIAL LIFE

When spring is in the air, don't get out and start to exercise like a fanatic. This can do more harm than good. Ask your medical practitioner or your personal trainer to work out the appropriate exercises and go about these exercises with enthusiasm. Exercise on a regular basis. Try not to skip any session. Once you have skipped a session it is easier to skip the next one, and before you know it, you are back in front of the television set. You must persevere and keep exercising. You will never regret it. It also gives you a sense of accomplishment if you can keep to your exercise schedule.

In this chapter, we also discuss the importance of a balanced social life but please remember that the world does not owe you a social life. Create social activities if there are none. We also discuss in some detail important travel tips to make those vacations abroad memorable ones—and not nightmares.

Chapter 11 YOU MUST (STILL) HAVE A PURPOSE IN LIFE

There must be a reason why you want to get out of bed in the morning. You should always have a purpose in life. You should still have a dream and be chasing after it no matter what your age.

Nobody is ever too old to have a dream. It does not matter what your dream is—as long as you still have one. It also does not matter whether your dream is little or big. Little or big is relative. What is big for one person might be little for another. Johann Wolfgang von Goethe advised "Dream no small dreams for they have no power to move the hearts of men."

If you do not already have one, get a good reason why you want to get out of bed in the morning. You must still have a purpose in life.

Chapter 12 PERSONAL HYGIENE

General good health is invaluable. If you could supplement good health with a well-groomed appearance and acceptable personal hygiene, you are a well on your way to enjoy a quality lifestyle.

In life there are many issues that can put a strain on our relationship with other people. Personal hygiene needs not be one of them!

Read about this important matter in this chapter and what you can do to improve your personal hygiene. It certainly is not rocket science.

EPILOGUE

If you should forget everything you read in this book, please remember this one truth. It is the wisdom of the late Father Frans Claerhout and should be everyone's prayer:

"GOD, YOU HAVE LOTS OF TIME—
I DON'T. HELP ME TO LIVE BEFORE I DIE."

BIBLIOGRAPHY

Drummer, Doris, Holidays RCI Group, *Autumn* (2010):

Editorial article, "Golden Rules of Goal Setting," *Mind Tools*, August 2009, http:/www.mindtools.com.

Klein, Shelly, *The Little Book of Senior Moments* (London: Michael O'Hara Books, 2008).

Pendleton, Winston K, *2121 Funny Stories and How to Tell Them*, (Missouri: The Bethany Press,1977).

In the course of writing this book, I consulted numerous general references, including Wikepedia, Who's Who, Biography Base and Brainy Quotes.